Sociology for Pharmacists
Second Edition

Also available from Taylor & Francis:

Pharmacy Practice
Edited by Kevin M.G. Taylor and Geoffrey Harding
ISBN 0-415-27158-4 (hardback) 0-415-27159-2 (paperback)

Textbook of Drug Design and Discovery (Third Edition)
Edited by Povl Krogsgaard-Larsen, Tommy Liljefors and Ulf Madsen
ISBN 0-415-28287-X (hardback) 0-415-28288-8 (paperback)

Drug Delivery and Targeting
Edited by Anya Hillery, Andrew Lloyd and James Swarbrick
ISBN 0-415-27198-3 (hardback)

Drug Misuse and Community Pharmacy
Edited by Janie Sheridan and John Strang
ISBN 0-415-28289-6 (hardback) 0-415-28290-X (paperback)

Pharmaceutical Biotechnology
Edited by Daan J.A. Crommelin and Robert D. Sindelar
ISBN 0-415-28500-3 (hardback) 0-415-28501-1 (paperback)

Introduction to Pharmacology
By Mannfred Hollinger
ISBN 0-415-28033-8 (hardback) 0-415-28034-6 (paperback)

Theory and Practice of Contemporary Pharmaceutics
Tapash K. Ghosh and Bhaskara R. Jasti
ISBN 0-415-28863-0 (hardback) 0-415-28864-9 (paperback)

Sociology for Pharmacists

An Introduction

Kevin Taylor

School of Pharmacy
University of London, UK

Sarah Nettleton

Department of Social Policy and Social Work
University of York, UK

and

Geoffrey Harding

St Bartholomew's and the Royal London School of Medicine and Dentistry,
Queen Mary, University of London, UK

Second Edition

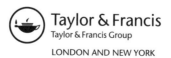

Taylor & Francis
Taylor & Francis Group

LONDON AND NEW YORK

First published 2003 by Taylor & Francis
11 New Fetter Lane, London EC4P 4EE

Simultaneously published in the USA and Canada
by Taylor & Francis Inc,
29 West 35th Street, New York, NY 10001

Taylor & Francis is an imprint of the Taylor & Francis Group

© 2003 By Kevin Taylor, Sarah Nettleton, Geoffrey Harding

Typeset in Palatino by Wearset Ltd, Boldon, Tyne and Wear
Printed and bound in Great Britain by TJ International Ltd, Padstow, Cornwall

Every effort has been made to ensure that the advice and information in this book is true and accurate at the time of going to press. However, neither the publisher nor the authors can accept any legal responsibility or liability for any errors or omissions that may be made. In the case of drug administration, any medical procedure or the use of technical equipment mentioned within this book, you are strongly advised to consult the manufacturer's guidelines.

British Library Cataloguing in Publication Data
A catalogue record for this book is available from the British Library

Library of Congress Cataloging in Publication Data
Taylor, Kevin, Ph.D.
  Sociology for pharmacists : an introduction / Kevin Taylor, Sarah Nettleton, Geoffrey Harding. – 2nd ed.
    p. ; cm.
  Rev. ed. of: Sociology for pharmacists / Geoffrey Harding, Sarah Nettleton, Kevin Taylor. 1990.
  Includes bibliographical references and index.
  1. Pharmacy—Social aspects. 2. Social medicine. 3. Sociology. [DNLM: 1. Sociology, Medical. 2. Pharmacy. WA 31 T243k 2003] I. Nettleton, Sarah, 1960– II. Harding, Geoffrey, 1954– III. Title.
RS92 .T39 2003
362.1′042—dc21

2003002015

ISBN 0-415-27487-7 (HB : alk. paper)
ISBN 0-415-27488-5 (PB : alk. paper)

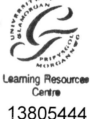

To our partners and children

Contents

Preface

This is the second edition of *Sociology for Pharmacists: An Introduction*, the first edition having been published in 1990. The philosophy of this revised book remains unchanged. It is written specifically for those studying or practising pharmacy who are newcomers to sociology; it introduces the key concepts of sociology and demonstrates their importance and application to pharmacy practice in the twenty-first century. Each chapter has been rewritten, updated and reformatted, and two chapters merged into one as we have endeavoured to ensure that this revised text reflects the changes in health care and pharmacy that have taken place in recent years.

We have written *Sociology for Pharmacists* in response to the recognition that sociology can contribute towards equipping pharmacists for their contemporary practice. The topics covered are by no means exhaustive; rather we have addressed those which we consider collectively, as sociologists, pharmacist and health care consumers, to be the most important.

The book begins with a short introductory section that highlights the changes and developments in society, pharmacy and pharmacy education which have resulted in the need to include sociology and social aspects of health care into the pharmacy under-graduate curriculum. In Chapter 1 we introduce the subject of sociology, key sociological concepts and theorists and outline the importance of a sociological perspective for effective pharmaceutical service delivery. In Chapter 2 we examine pharmacists' roles and activities in the context of the Nuffield Report on Pharmacy, the Pharmacy in a New Age (PIANA) initiative and recent and proposed changes in health policy. Sociological perspectives on the experience of health and illness, and illness behaviour are explored in Chapters 3 and 4, and we note that the presence of a symptom(s) alone does not necessarily result in an individual seeking help or treatment from a health professional, including a pharmacist. Chapters 5 and 6 demonstrate the ways in which health status and the experience of illness are influenced by such factors as gender, ethnicity, social class and employment status. In Chapter 7 we consider the occupational status of pharmacy from a sociological perspective and explore whether the status of pharmacy as a 'profession' is threatened or enhanced by actual and proposed changes in their activities. In Chapter 8 we consider the issues of health education and the pharmacists' role in health promotion and in ensuring that the public uses their medicines appropriately. Chapter 9 provides a brief introduction to methodological issues in sociological research and includes some guidance as to how these issues may be applied to research in the social aspects of pharmacy. Throughout the book reference is made to the sociology, medical and pharmacy literature and where appropriate readers are pointed towards additional reading.

We have written *Sociology for Pharmacists* primarily for pharmacy students, though it will also provide thought-provoking reading for pharmacists in community, hospital and academic practice. We have produced a sociology *for*, rather than a sociology *of* pharmacy, and envisage that the book will both inform practice and stimulate informed research into the social aspects of pharmacy practice.

Acknowledgements

We thank all those who have helped in the production of this book. In particular, we thank Maria Shew, Annie Cavanagh and Tess Andaya at the School of Pharmacy, University of London, for their expert help in the production of diagrams and tables. We are also very grateful to Linda Lisgarten, Michelle Wake and Mary McNicholl, in the library of the School of Pharmacy, for all their assistance in making sure we could access and appropriately cite many of the references used throughout the book.

Why a sociology for pharmacy?

The activities of pharmacists in primary and secondary care are subject to continuous change. Within secondary care, clinical and ward pharmacy have become prominent as concepts, with pharmacists increasingly integrated into the health care team, whilst at the same time pharmacists are able to specialise in, for instance, drug information, oncology, paediatrics and radiopharmacy. In primary care, recent decades have witnessed pharmacists' daily activities radically altered, so that activities such as compounding and formulating medicines have all but disappeared. As technological advances have made the dispensing of medicines a more routine task, how much of their time pharmacists spend on dispensing medicines is being called into question. At the same time the number of highly effective proprietary medicines available for sale from pharmacies, which were previously only available on prescription, has increased and is projected to increase still further. Moreover, in the near future pharmacists will be able to prescribe Prescription Only Medicines as supplementary prescribers. Taken together, these developments have led pharmacists to reassess what they do, and to promote themselves as health professionals, who in addition to being the acknowledged experts in medicines are capable of taking on greater responsibilities for patients' health status and the outcomes of drug treatment.

The time when pharmacy could be characterised as a lone pharmacist preparing and dispensing medicines, closeted away from the public, in the dispensary at the back of a shop has long gone. With the pharmaceutical manufacturing industry now producing medicinal products in packages complete with package inserts containing patient information suitable for dispensing direct to the consumer, and the employment of trained technical staff within pharmacies, even those pharmacists with the heaviest dispensing loads have more opportunity for embracing what has been referred to as the pharmacist's 'extended role'. This 'extended role' involves pharmacists interacting directly with the public, offering a range of services including diagnostic testing, health care advice, information, therapeutic recommendations, directions and instructions, in addition to ensuring that people receive the appropriate medication and understand how to use their medicines correctly. The allied concepts of pharmaceutical care and medicines management have been embraced, even if not wholly understood, by pharmacists and government to emphasise the positive contribution pharmacists, by their input to drug therapy, can make to patients' quality of life.

The undergraduate curriculum taught in UK schools of

pharmacy, extended by one year since 1997, has traditionally focused on the basic and applied sciences, including pharmaceutical chemistry, pharmaceutics, pharmacognosy, and pharmacology. In the 1970s and 1980s the curriculum in most schools was expanded to introduce the subject area of 'clinical pharmacy'. Clinical pharmacy draws on the knowledge of drugs and disease, as taught within a framework of the pharmaceutical sciences, and then relates this knowledge directly to the clinical requirements of patients; it includes pharmacokinetics, response to symptoms, disease aetiology and therapeutics.

The realisation within the pharmacy profession that its members were being increasingly called upon to respond to symptoms, give medical advice, 'counsel' patients and disseminate health education messages has resulted in the concept of 'pharmacy practice'. Pharmacy practice is an all-embracing term which describes a wide range of activities involved in the provision of pharmaceutical services. Consequently, it incorporates not only clinical pharmacy and the legal aspects of practice, but also various perspectives which assist in our understanding of the wider social context in which pharmaceutical services are delivered. Topics within the academic subject of pharmacy practice now include communication skills, medicines use, health economics, pharmacoepidemiology and pharmacovigilance.

Since pharmacists are increasingly assuming the role of 'health care professionals', rather than being solely dispensers of medicines and suppliers of medical appliances, pharmacy students require new skills as communicators, problem-solvers, reflexive thinkers, educators and advisers. 'Social and behavioural science' has been identified as having a significant contribution to make in the training of pharmacists. In the early 1980s an independent committee of inquiry was established under the aegis of the Nuffield Foundation, to closely examine all areas of the practice of pharmacy at that time. The findings of the Nuffield Inquiry, published in 1986, were a watershed in the historical development of pharmacy in the UK and were a precursor to many subsequent developments. Among its many recommendations, the so called 'Nuffield Report' advocated that behavioural science should be incorporated into the pharmacy undergraduate curriculum. The term 'behavioural science' denotes the scientific study of human behaviour and although it is most frequently associated with the discipline of psychology it implicitly includes other disciplines which study people and society, such as sociology and anthropology. In this book we are concerned specifically with the application of sociology to the practice of pharmacy. Sociology explains an individual's actions as a social phenomenon. That is to say, behaviour is explained and shaped by the society in which we live. For this reason, sociologists prefer to use the term 'social action' rather than 'behaviour'. Other areas included under the umbrella term 'behavioural science', for example social psychology and interpersonal communication, have been covered adequately in other texts and are beyond the remit of this book.

There is a fundamental need for pharmacists, and indeed for all health professionals, to have a sociologically informed approach to health care, since:

'Sociology demystifies the nature of health and illness, highlights the social causes of disease and death, exposes power-factors and ethical dilemmas in the production of health care, and either directly or indirectly helps to create a discerning practitioner who then becomes capable of more focussed and competent decision making' (Morrall, 2001).

The medical profession, earlier than pharmacy, recognised the importance of looking at health and illness from a sociological perspective and 'sociology as applied to medicine' has been routinely taught in nursing, medical and dental schools in the UK since the 1970s. The introduction of medical sociology into preclinical medical courses was a significant departure from those subjects previously taught in such courses. Prior to that time, teaching had tended to be based almost exclusively on detailed anatomical, histological and physiological studies of the tissues and organs of the body. It could similarly be argued that the teaching of pharmacy has traditionally concentrated on the 'drug entity', its derivation from plant and animal sources, its action on the body, its absorption, distribution, metabolism and elimination, its synthesis and chemical properties and formulation into dosage forms.

As schools of pharmacy and the Royal Pharmaceutical Society of Great Britain responded to the Nuffield Report, it became apparent that aspects of sociology should be incorporated into the pharmacy undergraduate curriculum in order to adequately prepare pharmacy students for their future practice. A working party of the Royal Pharmaceutical Society's Education Committee was instituted and its report (Working Party on Social and Behavioural Science, 1989) made thirteen recommendations with respect to the pharmacy degree course, the main recommendation being that, *'all schools of pharmacy should include teaching in the social science aspects of pharmacy, in the undergraduate pharmacy degree course'*. Subsequent pharmacy initiatives such as *Pharmacy in a New Age* (Royal Pharmaceutical Society of Great Britain, 1996), government policy as exemplified by the NHS Plan (Department of Health, 2000a, 2000b), and the evolution of pharmacists' roles – for instance, the advent of primary care pharmacists and pharmacist (supplementary) prescribing – mean that the awareness, by pharmacists, of the social dimension of health, illness and health care are more important than ever before. Indeed, the indicative pharmacy syllabus produced by the Royal Pharmaceutical Society of Great Britain, against which the degree programmes of British schools of pharmacy are accredited, includes a number of requirements relating to the need for pharmacy undergraduates to have an understanding of the social aspects of health and illness.

To meet these needs the remainder of this book provides an introduction to investigations of social practices of particular relevance to the practice of pharmacy.

REFERENCES

Department of Health (2000a) *Pharmacy in the Future – Implementing the NHS Plan*, London, Department of Health.

Department of Health (2000b) *The NHS Plan. A Plan for Investment. A Plan for Reform*, London, The Stationery Office.

Morrall, P. (2001) *Sociology and Nursing*, London, Routledge.

Nuffield Committee of Inquiry into Pharmacy (1986) *Pharmacy: a Report to the Nuffield Foundation*, London, Nuffield Foundation.

Royal Pharmaceutical Society of Great Britain (1996) *Pharmacy in a New Age: the New Horizon*, London, The Royal Pharmaceutical Society of Great Britain.

Working Party on Social and Behavioural Science (1989) *Report*, London, The Royal Pharmaceutical Society of Great Britain.

1 Sociology: An Introduction

Initially, the idea that pharmacists might usefully study sociology may appear a little odd. After all, pharmacists are surely concerned with drugs use, an activity which requires a sound understanding of the disciplines of physiology, pharmacology, pharmaceutical chemistry and pharmaceutics. Prescriptions need to be carefully checked and the therapeutic and adverse effects of medicines thoroughly understood. But of course, pharmacy is also 'people work'; drugs are dispensed to patients directly, or indirectly via informal carers, or other health professionals in the health care team. Furthermore, the general public seeks advice from pharmacists about medicines, treatments, alternative therapies and other aspects of their illness management and health maintenance. Pharmacists therefore need to be good communicators who are equipped with the appropriate skills for ensuring that they offer effective pharmaceutical care, and to this end there is now a range of texts available on communication and related skills for pharmacists. A sociological understanding of the issues of health, illness and health care can contribute to a deeper understanding of this people work. Sociologists have contributed to a better understanding of the actions and experiences of patients, the public, and health professionals who work within the health care system. This has resulted in a better appreciation of the nature of the relationships between health professionals and patients.

All of us have experience of health and illness. No doubt you will have been a patient, or you will have treated yourself when you felt ill, or you may have taken care of friends or relatives when they were unwell. This means that you will already have some knowledge and experience of the subject matter of this book. However, because the issues of health and illness are so familiar, it is difficult to distance ourselves from these and subject them to academic scrutiny. Indeed, a characteristic feature of sociology is that it often involves the systematic study of aspects of everyday life which are so familiar or routine that we do not give them a second thought. This means that it is all too easy to make assumptions about the way things are, and although they may appear to be 'obvious' they might in fact not be so. For instance, it is easy to assume that how we experience a disease and its symptoms are the consequence of biophysical changes in our bodies. However, social scientists have shown that the same physical symptoms can be interpreted in very different ways in different contexts, not only by patients but also by practitioners. For example, in Germany, low blood pressure is routinely treated by physicians as a disease, whereas in the UK this is not the case. Disease categories are not unambiguous descriptions of anatomical and physiological processes but are also imbued by the language, metaphors and values of a particular society (Sontag, 1978; Martin, 1994). They may also be contingent upon the nature of social and political relations in a given historical period. Consider hysteria for example, a disease classification that is now very rarely used by medical practitioners but which was common in the early part of the last century (Figlio, 1978). The diagnosis of disease is also affected by social factors. For example, a study undertaken in New Zealand found that out of 822 coronary bypass operations performed in 1983, only ten were carried out on the minority indigenous population – the Maori – even though the death rates from heart attack are significantly higher amongst that group (Pomare, 1998). This suggests that diagnostic procedures might not be purely objective but are in fact affected by social issues – the subject matter of sociology.

WHAT IS SOCIOLOGY?

Sociology is an academic discipline which makes use of a wide range of research methods to study society and social behaviour or social actions. Pharmacists, as a result of their school education and subsequent exposure to the pharmaceutical sciences as undergraduates tend to define themselves primarily as scientists. Science and 'scientific method' are part of their identity. On being introduced to sociology, students often approach it with preconceived ideas of it being 'soft', 'vague', 'undisciplined' and at times pretentious, peddling ideas that are little more than common sense. However, this presumption disregards the fact that sociology is a coherent discipline with a long tradition of applying a scientific perspective to social behaviour. Sociology is a science, generating and testing hypotheses, rigorously applying robust methods of empirical investigation to generate data whose analysis and interpretation leads to the formulation of theories. Sociology has amassed a body of knowledge from a variety of sources, employing a range of methodologies which may at first sight appear strange to pharmacists. These include social surveys, observations, analysis of language, and interviews (see Chapter 9). This knowledge has to be sufficiently robust to withstand exhaustive and widespread peer criticism, taking into account conflicting interpretations.

Throughout this book we will refer to a range of key sociological concepts which are outlined in Box 1.1. For clarity, these concepts have been reduced to their simplest terms, though we have sought to retain their essence and indicate in the text how they are likely to be important for the practice of pharmacy.

Social action is complex and we should not expect to unravel the complexity of the social world, and our behaviour within it, by simply applying 'common-sense' understandings. Bauman (1997) argues that sociology differs from common sense in the following respects:

1. *Responsible speech.* Sociological propositions are not founded on beliefs, but on corroborative evidence.
2. *Size of the field.* We understand common sense only from our individual perspective, i.e. it is partial knowledge. Sociology pursues a wider perspective – recognising the link between individual accounts and social processes of which individuals may be unaware.
3. *Making sense.* From a common-sense perspective, accounts of our actions are attributed back to someone – our actions are the intention of an individual. Sociologically, our actions are understood to be the result of our interdependency with our fellow members in society.
4. *Make the familiar strange.* Common sense is self-affirming: 'things are as they are', and 'people are as they are'. Sociology scrutinises the familiar in order to understand how common sense is as it is.

Agency:	Undetermined voluntary action by individuals
Norm:	Shared and expected social behaviour
Social role:	Expected actions associated with particular social positions
Social structure:	Recurring patterns of interrelationship between individuals or groups
Socialisation:	Acquiring and internalising the norms and values of a particular group
Society:	Configuration of cohesive social relationships within a particular group
Sociology:	Observation and analysis of societies

Box 1.1   Glossary of basic sociological concepts

The sociological imagination

In order to understand the processes that guarantee our ability to live cohesively together as members of a society, it is insufficient to take an individualistic point of view. That is, it is not sufficient to understand or explain people's actions solely through the behaviour of the individual or individuals concerned. Rather, it is necessary to take a wider social perspective and to understand the social forces that impinge, influence, or interact with the individual. These social forces are usually beyond the control of the individual. In many ways this forms the essence of sociological inquiry, which involves asking the question: what is the relationship between individual behaviour (or 'social action') and the social context (or 'social structure')? To develop an appreciation of the interaction of the individual in society is to come close to what the sociologist, C.W. Mills (1959) calls the 'sociological imagination'; that is, *'the urge to know the social and historical meaning of the individual in society'*.

An essential tool of the sociological imagination is the ability to distinguish between what Mills terms *'personal troubles of the milieu'* and *'the public issues of social structure'*. The complex relationship between individual social action and structured collective social action lies at the heart of the theoretical foundations of sociology and distinguishes it from the allied disciplines of social psychology and economics. We can consider society on two levels – the individual level (agency) and the collective level (structure). The sociologist aims to understand the interaction between these two. Let us take an example from Mills (1959):

'Consider marriage. Inside a marriage a man and a woman may experience personal troubles, but when the divorce rate during the first four years of marriage is 250 out of every 1,000 attempts, this is an indication of a structural issue having to do with the institution of marriage and family, and other institutions that bear upon them.'

Another example of an individual trouble that became a public issue is the controversy concerning the mumps, measles and rubella (MMR) vaccination in recent years. When a small group of individuals have personal worries over the triple vaccine, perhaps based on their beliefs about the potential harmful effects of vaccination *per se*, they may simply refuse it for their children. However, when a movement develops that questions the vaccine's safety, what once was a personal trouble becomes a public issue that impacts on public health and the public's relationship with health practitioners, medical 'experts' and the State.

How people act, think and behave is a result of the way in which they have been 'brought up'. In sociological terms, the relationship between our behaviour as both individuals and as members of society is termed 'agency/structure'. That is to say, the way we, as individuals, act is shaped by our social environment. In this sense we can never be free of the influences exerted on us by the social order to which we belong. Social rules and social norms have become internalised; that is, they become internal to the individual and are thus self-imposed rather than being subject to the control of others. Norms refer to actions that are expected or considered 'normal' in any given society.

We can see then, that individuals and the relationships between individuals are influenced by structural, i.e. broader social, economic and political circumstances. Sociology is not just about the collection of facts and information but is concerned primarily with understanding and interpretation. It can be confusing and daunting for those who are not used to this way of learning and thinking. What the sociologist studies is often familiar, i.e. it concerns our everyday activities. *'The sociologist does not look at a phenomenon that no one else is aware of, but he or she looks at the phenomenon in a different way'* (Berger, 1966).

SOCIOLOGICAL PERSPECTIVES AND THEIR APPLICATION TO PHARMACY

The boundaries of the discipline of sociology are difficult to define. This is in part because of the diverse and diffuse nature of its subject matter (namely people and society), but also because within the discipline of sociology there are many different approaches or perspectives – indeed there are many different types of sociology. While all the perspectives seek to understand how social structures interact with individual behaviours, they vary in terms of their level of analysis. Some are orientated towards micro-level issues, such as the actions and beliefs of individuals, while others illuminate macro-level issues that pertain to the way in which the 'structures' of society are organised. These would focus on questions such as: How are education or health care systems structured? How do economic systems work? What are the main social divisions within our society? Turner (1995) has usefully summarised three levels of analysis (individual, social and societal), and he illustrates the topics which might usefully be studied at these levels (see Table 1.1).

Working at the first level, sociologists examine people's accounts of their experiences of illness and how they maintain their health. The aim here is to illuminate aspects of everyday life from the perspective of the individual. Sociological perspectives orientated towards the individual level of analysis are the *'interpretive perspectives'* so called because they 'interpret' how people make sense of, and give meaning to, their lives or actions. Within interpretive approaches, attention is focused on how people interact at a face-to-face level; how they see their lives, make sense of their social circumstances and/or their physical symptoms. The key idea here is 'meaning', which refers to the way people make sense of what is happening to them. Sociologists therefore talk to and observe people to try and find out how they define their circumstances. To get an insight into how people see their situation, and why they see things as they do, is not however the same as

Level	Topic	Perspective
Individual	Lay knowledge of health, illness experience	Interpretive approaches
Social	Cultural categories of sickness	Structural-functionalism – sociology of roles, norms and deviance
Societal	Health care systems	Conflict perspectives, e.g. political economy

Table 1.1
Sociological perspectives and topics of health and illness (adapted from Turner, 1995)

saying that their view is 'correct'. Indeed, this is the case for any empirical sociological analysis – we can never access the unequivocal truth. Rather, in gaining a range of views of an issue, we can develop a fuller understanding. As Cuff *et al.* (1990) put it:

'Sociological perspectives merely provide us with ways of trying to understand the world; none of them has a built-in assurance that eternal and unshakable 'truth' will or can be provided.'

At the second level, sociologists use *'social perspectives'* to examine what society regards as sickness, illness or disease. Disease categories are not simply a reflection of biophysical processes within the body but are also the result of social considerations. It may seem ludicrous to us now, but until the early 1970s homosexuality was considered to be a sickness that had to be 'treated' because it was believed, by some, to be the result of physiological dysfunctions. Sickness and disease can therefore be understood as social as well as biological forms of deviance that are regulated and controlled by social institutions. Indeed, in our society one of the most powerful social institutions is Medicine. In our society, to be ill involves adopting a certain social role which involves obligations to get well and to seek expert help. Medical sociologists have called this the 'sick role', and this concept is discussed in Chapter 4. From this perspective (referred to as 'structural-functionalism') illness and disease prevent society functioning effectively, and consequently we have health professionals to help us get better when we are ill. From this perspective, illness is a form of social deviance and the medical profession exists, and is authorised, to help us get well. If we conform to the expected norms and obligations then the smooth running of society is maintained.

This view is not shared by all sociologists, and indeed an alternative *'societal perspective'* highlights 'conflict' rather than cohesion. The conflict perspective argues that the differential power and economic rewards that are given to those in social authority lead to social tension and conflict. Social order is maintained more through coercion than consensus. A variant of this perspective is the 'political economy approach' which highlights the ways in which socio-economic factors create and produce illness. For example, a major cause of illness in our society is poverty and material disadvantage. Another social determinant of illness that could be examined from within this perspective would be the ways in which the pharmaceutical industry has vested interests in 'creating' illness. For example, the industry would stand to gain from encouraging both the medical and pharmacy professions to treat mental health problems such as depression with drugs, rather than by using less invasive therapies. Thus, from this perspective those who are most powerful will have a vested interest in supporting the medical model of health and disease (Chapter 5) and the associated processes of medicalisation. Medicalisation is a sociological concept which refers to the ways in which more and more everyday life matters come to be dealt with by bio-medicine.

In this book it is not our intention to provide an exhaustive account of the full range of sociological perspectives and approaches. Indeed, it is inappropriate and unnecessary for pharmacy students to aspire to be sociologists in order to make sense of the impact of social influences on their professional activities. However, in order for readers to appreciate the context of key sociological concepts that recur throughout the book it is useful to provide a brief commentary on the historical emergence of the discipline of sociology and an overview of the theories generated by the key figures in the development of sociological perspectives.

Key theorists

The classical nineteenth-century sociological theorists whose ideas have shaped the discipline are Durkheim, Marx and Weber – the three so-called 'founding fathers' of sociology. To make sense of their theories it is important to first consider the social context in which their ideas were developed.

Two historical revolutions were instrumental in setting the scene for the emergence of sociology as a discipline – the French Revolution of 1789 and the European-wide Industrial Revolution of the nineteenth and early twentieth centuries. Such was the impact of these revolutions that social life underwent a profound and rapid change, the like of which had not been previously experienced. This rapid social transformation led to the development of systematic enquiries into how society could undergo such change. The Industrial Revolution was responsible for increasing the production of goods and services on a hitherto inconceivable scale and changed a way of life that had endured for millennia. As has been pointed out by one of the most influential contemporary sociologists, *'the Englishman of 1750 was closer in material things to Caesar's legionnaires than to his own great-grandchildren'* (Giddens, 1986).

Émile Durkheim (1858–1917)

Durkheim's contribution to sociology has been a theory of how social order is maintained and cohesive social relations are established. He believed the task for sociology was to study what he termed 'social facts', with the same objectivity as natural scientists make their observations. Social facts were forces such as shared belief systems, which operated on individuals in a coercive way. As these social facts changed, so too did the forces they exerted on individuals, resulting in new forms of social action. His most celebrated work was a study of suicide (originally published in 1897). Durkheim set out to show empirically that changes in the rates of suicide – the most individual of acts – could be linked to social facts. Various forms of suicide were shown to be related to social facts – not to an individual's mind-set at a particular time. For example, a war would give rise to increased rates of *altruistic suicide* – soldiers deliberately sacrificing their lives to save their comrades. Box 1.2 gives an example of how Durkheim's concept of social forces operates in the context of pharmacy.

Box 1.2 An example of the application to pharmacy of Durkheim's thinking on the social order

The functions of pharmacists include contributing to legitimating an individual's sickness, by diagnosing illness, supplying medication and referral to a general practitioner. By expediting people's 'flight into health' and helping to ensure that prescribed medicines are taken in accordance with the prescriber's wishes, pharmacists ensure people overcome their sickness and return to their regular productive activities, thus maintaining the social order.

Karl Marx (1818–83)

Marx, although considered to be more an economist than a sociologist, was responsible for developing what is known as a Marxist perspective. This draws on a theory of capitalist society which, put simply, argues that people, of necessity, express themselves productively; that is, in order to live we need to produce goods to meet our basic needs – food, clothing and shelter. Throughout history, Marx argues, this otherwise natural form of expression has never been freely allowed to develop. There has always been an element of exploitation in which one group (the ruling class) seeks to take advantage of other groups (the working class) through perhaps enslaving them, controlling the land on which they live, or, as in capitalist societies, exploiting workers by expropriating the goods produced and providing in return a limited wage. Central to Marx's theory of capitalism is a sense that the social order, rather than being held together by external forces such as a shared morality, is coercively held together by an ideology which functions to preserve the oppressive character of society and the capitalist economy's mode of production. Today, Marxism is a rather outmoded theory, but its more modern form is the political economy perspective which we have discussed above. Box 1.3 gives an example of how a Marxist perspective might be applied to pharmacy.

Max Weber (1864–1920)

Weber sought to establish a theory of rationalisation within industrialised societies. For Weber, bureaucracy was the classic form of

Box 1.3 An example of a Marxist perspective on the functioning of the pharmaceutical industry

> Medicines are an internationally traded commodity that depend on the creation of a market for their consumption. A Marxist perspective may propose that the pharmacist's role in promoting drug consumption serves the interests of large pharmaceutical manufacturing corporations rather than the general population. Large pharmaceutical companies have a vested interest in defining so called 'health problems' to which their product is an 'answer'. To do so distracts attention from the underlying socio-economic basis for much illness. For instance, the supply/purchase of drugs to deal with the symptoms of stress serves to detract from the underlying causes of stress which, it could be argued, have an economic and social basis.

rationalisation. The industrialised world was, for Weber, the very epitome of modernisation, as the social order depends for its smooth existence on technical efficiency – a world dominated by the principles of efficiency, calculability and predictability. Unlike Marx, who believed that the inherent contradictions in the social relations of capitalism would ultimately result in its replacement by a utopian ideal state without large-scale class divisions (i.e. communism), Weber believed there was no new social order waiting in the wings. The tenets of rationality are so closely stitched into the fabric of the modern industrial capitalist world that individuals are unable to resist them. Instead, Weber argues we must resign ourselves to a world ordered by bureaucracy, creating, in Weber's own words, an 'iron cage' from which we cannot escape. Box 1.4 presents an example of how Weber's concept of rationality and bureaucracy is applicable to pharmacy.

Box 1.4 An example of Weber's theories of bureaucratisation and rationalisation within pharmacy

> Community pharmacies increasingly function as part of large bureaucratic structures as multiple chains of pharmacies and in-store supermarket pharmacies proliferate. Bureaucracies seek to enhance productivity and profits by instituting rationalised and routinised processes. The activities of workers are inevitably broken down into smaller, calculable components whilst standardised work procedures and technology, designed to increase productivity, are introduced wherever possible. Such developments, it can be argued, are the antithesis of traditional professional activity which places great store on mystical skills and autonomy of action.

Modernity – the 'old world order'

Durkheim, Marx and Weber shared a common interest in attempting to understand how the social order is maintained by applying scientific principles of analysis. They were writing in a historical period which is often referred to as 'modernity'. A feature of academic thinking during this time was that objective (as opposed to interpretive or subjective) knowledge is uncovered. By the rigorous application of scientific principles, objective 'truths' emerge. Key to the modernist approach is the assumption that different forms of knowledge exist and are hierarchical – at the very pinnacle is scientific knowledge, generated by science, while common-sense knowledge or knowledge based on experience alone is relegated as being either self-evident or subjective knowledge (with the associated connotation of being less valid). This view of knowledge has been challenged by contemporary theorists. Many now argue that experiential knowledge is undoubtedly different but no less important than scientific knowledge.

Post-modernity

A post-modern stance is one which maintains that objective knowledge, such as that generated through scientific enquiry, is not necessarily qualitatively more valid than other forms of knowledge, and that scientific 'knowledge' is, like all knowledge, socially constructed rather than passively discovered. Hence, whereas the scientific knowledge base of say pharmacognosy represents nature 'giving up its secrets' regarding the medicinal properties of plants, it is now also possible to 'know' the medicinal properties of plants by other than scientific trails and experimentation, as with, for example, 'experiencing' the medicinal properties of essential oils.

Scientific knowledge, medicines use and the dilemmas of choice

Since Durkheim, Marx and Weber laid the foundations for sociology, the discipline of sociology has developed considerably. The world we inhabit has changed beyond recognition since the early twentieth century, and while issues such as social inequalities and the distribution of power in society have not undergone any marked change, Western societies have become evermore complex. With this increased level of complexity have come new challenges. In terms of pharmacy, one only need consider the revolutions in drug therapy, particularly in the past fifty years, and more recently the ready availability of powerful medications over the counter from community pharmacies. The developments in the pharmaceutical sciences which have given the public access to these powerful drugs, whether they are prescribed or purchased, highlight the fact that in life today, more than ever before, individuals are involved in managing and assessing health-related risks. Whilst the prevalence of risks to our health has not quantitatively increased, we are increasingly made aware, as a result of science and technology, of apparently 'new' risks such as environmental pollution, global warming, BSE and genetically modified foodstuffs. Moreover we are expected to assess and manage such risks ourselves by 'doing our bit', rather than relying exclusively on others, the so-called 'experts', to do so on our behalf. So prevalent is the idea of having to assess and manage risks in our everyday life that the term *Risk Society* has been coined (Beck, 1992). One tenet of the Risk Society is that all our actions involve calculating their associated risk. Whatever we do, we do on the basis of projected outcomes. In recent times, for instance, many parents have had to balance the risk of immunising their children with the risks associated with non-immunisation. Assessing risks is clearly evident for individuals with regard to their consumption of medicines. For instance, a calculation of risk is involved in not taking a prescribed medicine (e.g. 'my body will become resistant to antibiotics if I take too many') which is weighed against taking the medicine (e.g. 'I will not get better unless I take all the prescribed antibiotics'). Similarly, with increasing deregulation of medicines which previously could only be accessed by a prescription to their being openly available over the counter, the purchase of these medicines involves the purchaser in a risk assessment, given that at the least they might not be efficacious and therefore a waste of money, but at worst could cause harm. Pharmacists, each time they sell such a medicine are also required to make a risk assessment. Careful questioning of a prospective purchaser will inform a pharmacist's decision regarding whether to supply the product, yet all risk cannot be eliminated: what if the purchaser is not telling the truth, is pregnant, is allergic to the medication, or has an underlying undiagnosed medical condition?

Pharmacy in contemporary society

Pharmacy is undergoing rapid change and development, with pharmacists being encouraged to take on new roles, including those of community- and hospital-based health advisers and promoters, and indeed medicine prescribers. Taking on these new roles presents pharmacists with a number of difficulties. For instance, not all individuals will respond to symptoms in the same way, not everyone has faith in orthodox medicine, and the need to seek treatment is not necessarily a top priority for everyone, competing as it does with other factors such as work and family commitments, or difficulties of transport and mobility.

Appreciating the social dimensions of health and illness, together with the application of their specialist knowledge of drugs and drug therapy, will ensure that the advice and/or treatment offered by pharmacists is appropriate to an individual patient's particular needs. A sociological perspective applied to pharmacy provides an insight into an individual's responses to illness and medication use through an appreciation of health beliefs which are shaped by the social context. The concern here is not with a psychological interpretation of how an individual's particular mind-set explains their behaviour. The focus, from a sociologically informed perspective, is on the way in which social forces – collective beliefs, values and attitudes – act upon individuals, and in so doing account for the motivations and constraints that influence their use, misuse and non-use of medicines and health care services. The purpose of the remainder of this book is not to transform pharmacists into sociologists but rather to equip present and future pharmacists with some basic concepts and insights drawn from sociology which may be applied to their daily practice. This position stands midway between Strauss's (1957) distinction of the 'Sociology of Medicine' (sociologists examining medicine and medical practice from sociological presuppositions) and 'Sociology in Medicine' (sociologists working with bio-medicine's presuppositions). What we have endeavoured to produce, within this book, is a sociology *for* pharmacy – a blend of both sociological concepts and the empirical realities of pharmacy in the twenty-first century.

SUMMARY

- Sociology is an academic discipline which applies a range of research methodologies to systematically study modern societies
- An adequate understanding of society is facilitated by a 'sociological imagination' – that is, the ability to appreciate the interaction between an individual's 'personal troubles' and society's 'public issues'
- Sociology comprises a number of perspectives and approaches which pertain to three levels of analysis – the individual, social and societal
- The foundations of sociological theory can be traced to social theorists in the nineteenth century – these include Durkheim, Marx and Weber
- Contemporary society is characterised by rapid social and technological change, and these changes directly influence the work of pharmacists.

FURTHER READING

Barry, A.M. and Yuill, C. (2002) *Understanding Health: A Sociological Introduction*, London, Sage.

Beck, U. (1992) *Risk Society: Towards a New Modernity*, London, Sage.

Bilton, T., Bonnett, K., Jones, P., Lawson, T., Skinner, D., Stanworth, M. and Webster, A. (2002) *Introductory Sociology* (4th edn), London, Palgrave.

Giddens, A. (2001) *Sociology* (4th edn), Cambridge, Polity Press.

REFERENCES

Bauman, Z. (1997) Thinking sociologically. In: A. Giddens (ed.) *Sociology: Introductory Readings* (2nd edn), Cambridge, Polity Press, pp. 12–18.

Beck, U. (1992) *Risk Society: Towards a New Modernity*, London, Sage.

Berger, P. (1966) *Invitation to Sociology: a Humanistic Perspective*, Harmondsworth, Penguin.

Cuff, E.C., Sharrock, W.W. and Francis, D.W. (1990) *Perspectives in Sociology*, London, Routledge.

Figlio, K. (1978) Chlorosis and chronic disease in nineteenth-century Britain: the social constitution of somatic illness in a capitalist society. *International Journal of Health Services*, 8, 589–617.

Giddens, A. (1986) *Sociology: A Brief but Critical Introduction* (2nd edn), London, Macmillan.

Martin, E. (1994) *Flexible Bodies: The Role of Immunity in American Culture from the Days of Polio to the Age of AIDS*, Boston, Beacon Press.

Mills, C.W. (1959) *The Sociological Imagination*, New York, Oxford University Press.

Morrall, P. (2001) *Sociology and Nursing*, London, Routledge.

Pomare, E. (1988) Groups with special health care needs. *New Zealand Medical Journal*, 101, 297–308.

Sontag, S. (1978) *Illness as a Metaphor*, New York, Farrar, Straus and Giroux.

Strauss, R. (1957) The nature and status of medical sociology, *American Sociological Review*, 22, 200–204.

Turner, B.S. (1995) *Medical Power and Social Knowledge*, London, Sage.

2 Contemporary Practice of Pharmacy

INTRODUCTION

In this chapter we have not attempted to provide a detailed historical account of the development of pharmacy from its earliest history through to the present day (a brief outline of the history of pharmacy is presented in Chapter 7), nor have we provided an exhaustive account of pharmacists' day-to-day activities. Rather, we show how the activities of pharmacists have evolved over recent years and that pharmacists are now expected, by both the public and the State, to provide a wider range of services than in the past.

In 1983, a major independent review of the pharmacy profession was undertaken. The Committee of Inquiry into Pharmacy, commonly referred to as the 'Nuffield Inquiry', was an independent investigation into the practice of pharmacy in Great Britain. The inquiry received submissions from a wide range of sources, including pharmacists from all branches of pharmacy and representatives of the British Medical Association, the Consumers' Association, and societies representing a broad spectrum of other health care professionals. The terms of reference for the inquiry were *'to consider the present and future structure of the practice of pharmacy in its several branches and its potential contribution to health care and to review the education and training of pharmacists accordingly'*. The report of the inquiry, published in 1986, has become known as the Nuffield Report (Nuffield Committee of Inquiry, 1986). Ninety-six conclusions and recommendations were contained in the Report, relating to community, hospital and industrial pharmacy, undergraduate, postgraduate and continuing education, pharmacy practice research and the Pharmaceutical Society of Great Britain. Many of the developments that have occurred in pharmacy in subsequent years can be traced back to the recommendations contained in the Nuffield Report, which highlighted the ways in which pharmacists' skills might be more appropriately utilised.

THE PHARMACY WORKFORCE

Currently there are approximately 40,000 registered pharmacists in Great Britain, the majority working in community or hospital pharmacy: 62 per cent practice in the community, 17 per cent practice in hospital pharmacies and 5 per cent work in industry (Table 2.1).

The traditional image of a pharmacist, often still perpetrated by the media, is of a white-coated, middle-aged white male. However, the reality is that pharmacists are nowadays more likely to be women as men and increasingly may come from an ethnic minority. In recent decades there has been a marked increase in

Principal occupation	Male		Female	
	Number	%	Number	%
Community	11,674	68.0	10,645	56.7
Hospital	1,625	9.4	4,354	23.2
Industry	969	5.6	735	3.9
Wholesale	67	0.4	16	0.1
Teaching	203	1.2	74	0.4
Other pharmacy	577	3.4	792	4.2
Non-pharmacy	415	2.4	368	2.0
No paid employment	824	4.8	664	3.5
Working (sector unknown)	835	4.9	1,118	6.0
Missing data	1,953	–	1,559	–
Total	**19,142**	**100**	**20,325**	**100**

Table 2.1 Principal occupation of pharmacists registered with the Royal Pharmaceutical Society of Great Britain in 2001 (reproduced with permission from Hassell *et al.*, 2002)

the proportion of women pharmacists. In the UK, 51.5 per cent of the pharmacy workforce are women (Table 2.1) compared to less than 20 per cent in the mid-1960s (Hassell and Symonds, 2001) and women represent the large majority of those practising in the hospital sector. This reflects the fact that in recent years the majority of entrants into Schools of Pharmacy have been women, with the proportion of women registering as pharmacists increasing from 53 per cent in 1975 to 68 per cent in 1991 (Hassell *et al.*, 1998). Studies have also indicated that after having children, an increased proportion of women work in community pharmacy, often choosing to work part-time. Indeed, 75 per cent of part-time pharmacists are women (Hassell *et al.*, 2002). This trend towards a situation where the majority of pharmacists are women accompanies an increase in the representation of ethnic minorities within the pharmacy workforce. In 1975, 15 per cent of those qualifying as pharmacists in the UK came from an ethnic minority. By 1991, ethnic minorities comprised 23 per cent of qualifying pharmacists (Hassell *et al.*, 1998). This compares with a total ethnic minority population within the UK of 5.5 per cent. In 1998, 44 per cent of applicants to schools of pharmacy in the UK were from ethnic minorities (Hassell and Symonds, 2001).

HOSPITAL PHARMACY

Until the mid-1960s, hospital pharmacists, like their colleagues working in the community, were engaged mainly in the compounding and dispensing of medicines. As in community pharmacies, the majority of medicines dispensed from hospital pharmacies are now manufactured by the pharmaceutical industry. Only specialised items, such as certain sterile products which cannot be supplied by industry, are manufactured 'in house'. As more and more potent drug substances with narrow therapeutic index come onto the market, the potential for serious medication errors, adverse drug reactions and drug interactions has increased. Consequently, the need has arisen for the pharmacists to play a more active and direct role in the provision of pharmaceutical services within hospitals. This has resulted in the concept of 'ward pharmacy'. Pharmacists at the ward level may be involved in decisions regarding patient medication at the pre-prescription stage, working alongside physicians, supplying them with pharmaceutical and therapeutic information and assisting in the selection and use of the appropriate medication. An Audit Commission study of medicines management within NHS hospitals (Audit Commission, 2001) recommended that pharmacists be integrated into the clinical team, recognising that *'Pharmacists are experts in pharmacology and bringing them closer to the patient improves the quality of care and reduces costs'*. The report recognised that, as in the community, hospital pharmacists have a role to play in ensuring patients receive their medicines appropriately, indicating that typically between one-fifth and one-quarter of in-patient prescription charts are amended by pharmacists. In addition to their activities at ward level, hospital pharmacists are now involved in the supply of drugs (to inpatients and out-patients), stock control, and pharmacist-led clinics such as anti-coagulation clinics and prescription monitoring. In addition, pharmacists may discuss treatment with patients prior to and upon discharge from hospital which can result in benefits in terms of medication management, reduced readmission rates and reduced wastage of patients' own medicines (Brookes *et al.*, 2000). They may also supply drug information to doctors, nurses and other members of the primary health care team, and where appropriate to patients and their relatives.

There is scope for a degree of specialisation within hospital pharmacy. Hence pharmacists may specialise in, for example, therapeutic drug monitoring, radio-pharmacy, oncology, drug information, production, quality assurance and quality control.

COMMUNITY PHARMACY

The Nuffield Report stated that *'Pharmacists have a unique and vital role to play in the provision of health care to the community'*. This report and later government White Papers on health care have suggested an extension of pharmacists' activities beyond what might be considered their traditional role: the dispensing of pre-scribed medicines. This expansion of the community pharmacist's role, along with the National Pharmaceutical Association's 'Ask your Pharmacist' campaign, the distribution of health promotion material from pharmacies, reclassification of prescription only medicines such that they are now available from pharmacies, and the advertising of medicines to the public which are only available from pharmacies, has raised the profile of community pharmacists as a readily accessible provider of health care, and a 'first port of call' in seeking medical advice and treatment. During 1995 and 1996, the Royal Pharmaceutical Society of Great Britain ran a consultation process with its membership. The so-called Pharmacy in a New Age (PIANA) initiative sought to identify how the pharmacy should develop to meet public health needs (see pp. 27–28).

A relatively recent development has been the increasing number of pharmacists working within GP practices, often on a part-time or sessional basis. These have come to be known as primary care pharmacists and represent an increased integration of pharmacists into the primary care team. For a review of the activities of such pharmacists, readers are referred to Jesson and Wilson (1999). They have highlighted the key areas of activity for primary care pharmacists, which are outlined in Box 2.1. Such pharmacists have a major role in managing prescribed medication costs through medication reviews for individual patients. Research has shown that these medication reviews, when conducted by a pharmacist, can generate considerable savings for primary care trusts (Zermansky *et al.*, 2001).

Box 2.1 Key areas of activity for primary care pharmacists (Jesson and Wilson, 1999)

1. Cost-effective prescribing
2. Medicines management
3. Education
4. Patient contact

DISPENSING OF PRESCRIBED MEDICATION

It has been estimated that in 1999, around 530 million NHS prescription items were dispensed in the UK, working out at about ten prescription items per person per year (Department of Health, 2000a). In England and Wales, in the year up to March 2001, 10,471 community pharmacies dispensed 561.8 million NHS prescription items (Pharmaceutical Journal, 2001). Thus, the average community pharmacy dispenses approximately 4,400 items per month. The main function of the pharmacist, as perceived by both the public and the State, is at present the dispensing of prescribed medicines, and this activity takes the greatest part of their time (Rutter *et al.*, 1998). For independent pharmacies, remuneration for dispensing prescribed medication remains the major component of their income.

Currently, virtually all prescriptions written by general practitioners are dispensed from pharmacies (the remainder, about 5 per cent, being accounted for by dispensing doctors). Pharmacists have an important function in ensuring that patients receive the appropriate medication, that they store it correctly, and are aware of how to take or use it properly. This is particularly important in the light of surveys which have indicated an error rate of between 3 per cent and 10 per cent in prescriptions written by general practitioners (Jones, 1978; Neville et al., 1989; Shah et al., 2001). One study monitored the prescriptions generated by eight doctors in a single practice over a period of three months (Neville et al., 1989). Of the 15,916 prescriptions generated, 504 (3 per cent) contained some sort of prescribing error. Sixty-two had 'trivial' errors; that is, those which were technically incorrect but in which the error was of a very minor nature, or the prescriber's intentions were obvious, for instance spelling errors. A further 273 had 'minor' errors which involved the pharmacist in making a professional decision but which did not require a consultation with the prescriber – for example, ordering of an inappropriate pack size of a dermatological product. One hundred and sixty-nine prescriptions had 'major' errors, such that the pharmacist needed to contact the prescriber for clarification – for example, if the prescription was illegible or incomplete. A later study of prescriptions written by twenty-three general practitioners in three practices over a period of two months (Shah et al., 2001) confirmed the earlier findings and demonstrated that the error rate varied significantly between prescribers in different general practices and that the error rate was higher for handwritten prescriptions (10.2 per cent) than for those that were computer-generated (7.9 per cent).

A comparable situation exists in secondary care. A recent study in a London teaching hospital revealed that 1.5 per cent of hospital prescriptions written by doctors were discovered by pharmacists to contain errors, approximately a quarter of which were likely to cause significant harm (Dean et al., 2002).

Pharmacists and prescribers share the responsibility for ensuring that the patients receive the appropriate dispensed medicines and are advised on their correct use. This was highlighted in 1982 by the so-called 'Migril case' in which it was ruled in the High Court that the pharmacist and the prescriber were equally liable for a prescribed, and subsequently dispensed, overdose of the drug Migril (ergotamine tartrate) which resulted in a patient developing gangrene in both feet. In this case the pharmacist, who admitted negligence, was found to be 45 per cent responsible for the error and the prescriber 55 per cent responsible. The judge stated that the pharmacist owed a duty of care to the patient to ensure that the drug was correctly prescribed (Applebe and Wingfield, 2001). In a similar case in which a family suffered adverse effects as a result of being prescribed daily instead of weekly doses of the anti-malarial drug chloroquine, the pharmacist and doctor were deemed to be responsible in the ratio of 40:60 respectively (Pharmaceutical Journal, 1989). Consequently, it is in the pharmacist's interest as well as the patient's that procedures exist and are followed within the pharmacy to ensure that the patient receives the appropriate medication, suitably labelled, and that the patient will use that medication correctly.

Nowadays the majority of prescribed medicines dispensed by pharmacists do not need to be manufactured from their constituent ingredients. Indeed, many pharmacists will no longer undertake the most basic manufacturing procedures, rather arranging for medicines requiring compounding to be produced by a 'specials' manufacturer. Over the past decade there has also been an increasing tendency for medicines manufactured by the pharmaceutical industry to be supplied in packages ready for 'original pack' or 'patient pack' dispensing, whereby a medicine can be supplied to a patient without the pharmacist having to count dosage units. Patient information leaflets (PILs) are included in the packs, providing the patient with information which might once have been supplied by the pharmacist. Thus, pharmacists are spending less time in measuring and counting medicines than in the very recent past. The introduction of computers into pharmacies and the availability of appropriate software have also markedly reduced the time spent by pharmacists on activities such as labelling of medicines and stock control, whilst corresponding computer-based technology in prescribers' surgeries reduces the potential for prescribing errors and even results in the production of legible prescription forms!

Taken together, these developments have considerably reduced the time required to dispense prescribed medicines. Moreover, most pharmacies employ trained dispensing assistants/technicians who are more than adequately equipped to perform the routine technical aspects of medicines dispensing over which the pharmacist exercises supervisory control. Additionally, in the future pharmacists may not be required to supervise every medicine dispensed, as is currently the case. Indeed, the recent discussion paper, *Pharmacy Workforce in the New NHS* (Department of Health, 2002), states that:

'The modern pharmacist's professional role is not primarily to undertake detailed supervision of the dispensing and sale of medicines. Experience in the hospital sector has shown that these tasks can be delegated to suitably trained staff.'

The reduction in the time which pharmacists need to be actively involved in dispensing medicines has created the possibility for them to develop further their professional activities. From the pharmacists' viewpoint this may be particularly important, as when their key roles are seen to be 'technical' and capable of routinisation they may no longer be able to claim the privileged occupational status they currently enjoy (see Chapter 7).

George Ritzer, an American sociologist, has argued that contemporary society is characterised by the process of rationalisation, a process originally outlined in the work of Max Weber (see Chapter 1). Ritzer has coined the term 'McDonaldisation' (Ritzer, 2000) to illustrate how the policies and practices required for the optimal, efficient, routinised production and delivery of fast food are evident in other organisations, including the health care sector. Ritzer has outlined four dimensions of the rationality inherent to McDonaldisation which are outlined in Box 2.2.

Box 2.2 The four dimensions of rationality inherent to McDonaldisation

Efficiency:	Optimal methods for completing tasks are employed
Predictability:	Production processes are organised to guarantee the uniformity of products and standardised outcomes
Calculability:	Outcomes are assessed quantitatively, i.e. there is an emphasis on quantity rather than quality
Control:	Since people are inherently unpredictable and inefficient, control is achieved either through automation or de-skilling of the workforce

The process of rationalisation applied to pharmacy, focuses on streamlining the process of delivering pharmaceutical services. Pharmacists' unique skills and knowledge vie with the overarching expediency of developing evermore rational means of delivering services. McDonaldisation is evident in all branches of pharmacy, but most obviously in the community sector. Technological advances within the pharmaceutical industry, computer technology in pharmacies and the progressive domination of large multiple chain and supermarket pharmacies (the number of independent pharmacies – chains of five or less – in England and Wales fell by 27.5 per cent between 1991 and 2001: Pharmaceutical Journal, 2001) ensure that Ritzer's four dimensions of rationality are clearly evident (Harding and Taylor, 2000). Future developments such as electronic transfer of prescriptions and mail order pharmacy, together with the introduction of robotic dispensing, may extend this process yet further.

Efficiency

Products and services are standardised where possible. For example, patient pack medicines ensure rapid, efficient processing. A production line approach to prescription filling reminiscent of car manufacturing is adopted. This requires a number of technicians each completing just a small part of the overall process to ensure speed of service and rapid throughput of customers.

Predictability

Multiple pharmacies standardise their services, products and pack sizes, so that all their outlets offer identical 'experiences'. Own-brand medicines are available in all outlets. These outlets are invariably of a uniform design and staffed by uniformed individuals well drilled in the company ethos (i.e. they are subject to a corporate socialisation process), and company protocols and procedures are designed to ensure consistency of service.

Calculability

Many large pharmacies trade in commodities of which medicines are but one among a wide range of other, often lifestyle-related, products. These products are marketed on the basis of having low-cost value, rather than an emphasis on their quality and efficacy. For instance, with the recent abolition of 'Resale Price Maintenance', which fixed the price of over-the-counter medicines, these products may now be sold on the basis of price, resulting in 'three for the price of two', and 'buy one get one free' offers.

Control

Skilled activities are minimised as operatives undertake simple, clearly defined tasks in accordance with written procedures. Control is exercised over consumers by their exposure to corporate advertising, which encourages familiarity with own-brand products. Also, computer technology is used wherever possible – for example to generate labels and information leaflets, order replacement stock and for drug information. Robotic dispensing, already employed within the hospital sector, is also likely to be introduced into community pharmacy where cost-effective.

Taken together these developments can be said to represent the de-skilling of pharmacy and present challenges to pharmacists' ability to claim that their work is special – i.e. that of a professional – and as such enable them to reap benefits in terms of status, remuneration and autonomy of action (see Chapter 7).

PHARMACISTS' ACTIVITIES NOT DIRECTLY RELATED TO DISPENSING

A community pharmacy's NHS remuneration is largely dependent on the number of items dispensed. This tying of remuneration to dispensing activity is seen by many as hampering opportunities for pharmacy to develop. The Royal Pharmaceutical Society, through its initiatives such as Pharmacy in a New Age (PIANA), launched in October 1995, has sought to promote pharmacists' activities, additional to dispensing, through concepts such as pharmaceutical care and medicines management. Following a period of extensive consultation with its membership, resulting from the PIANA initiative, the RPSGB (1996) published its *Pharmacy in a New Age: The New Horizon* document, which identified four key areas in which pharmacists should be involved (Box 2.3).

Box 2.3 Key areas for pharmacy involvement resulting from the PIANA initiative

1. The management of prescribed medicines
2. The management of chronic conditions
3. The management of common ailments
4. The promotion and support of healthy lifestyles

With the increasing emphasis on pharmacists undertaking activities not associated with dispensing medicines, the possibility of pharmacist prescribing in the near future (see pp. 31–32), and the likelihood that the rules necessitating that pharmacists supervise the dispensing of all prescriptions will be relaxed (Department of Health, 2002), it seems that the future will witness a diminishing of the time pharmacists spend directly involved in medicine supply. Meanwhile, additional activities will be adopted, promoted and imposed.

The pharmacist's 'extended role'

A pharmacist's undergraduate and pre-registration training ensures that they have extensive pharmacological, pharmaceutical and clinical knowledge relating to drug compounds and medicines. Moreover, pharmacists are required to acquire and develop pharmaceutical skills unique among health professionals. These skills equip pharmacists to be more than just dispensers of medicines.

At the point of handing over a dispensed medicine, pharmacists have an opportunity to reiterate and reinforce the prescribers' instructions and, where appropriate, give additional advice and information. By reinforcing the prescriber's instructions, already provided on the medicine's label, pharmacists may facilitate the likelihood of adherence (compliance) of patients with the prescribed drug regimen. Moreover, since pharmacies are readily accessible in most communities, pharmacists are available to provide more general health care advice. Such advice may involve the diagnosis and treatment of minor illness and, where necessary, the referral of patients to a general practitioner. Advice may go beyond illness and medicines and encompass advice regarding diet, smoking cessation, complementary therapies, etc. In addition to providing health advice to the public, studies have indicated that a majority of community pharmacists are consulted by general practitioners and other health professionals, including dentists, midwives, nurses and health visitors.

The increased availability of potent drugs, the complex nature of modern drug therapy, and the occurrence of iatrogenic (drug-caused) disease ensure that pharmacists, because of their specialist knowledge of drug substances, have a crucial and indeed unique contribution to make to health care. Moreover, the public is increasingly exercising its power as the consumer of health care resources and services (see Chapter 4). The public's expectations of health professionals have risen and therefore these professions must be prepared to offer a high-quality service and, if required, a competitive range of services. The services offered by pharmacists in addition to the traditional dispensing activities have become known as the pharmacists' 'extended role'. The government's Green and White Papers on Primary Health Care (DHSS, 1986, 1988), which built on the findings and recommendations of the earlier Nuffield Inquiry, outlined some of the features of the 'extended role' of the pharmacist and determined the likely future development of pharmaceutical services. The 'extended role' *per se* has not actually been comprehensively defined, however Box 2.4 outlines those components which were originally suggested in the Nuffield Report and have gained general acceptance since. To these, other features have been added – as will more in due course.

Advising patients on minor ailments, recommending treatments and 'counselling' patients on the correct way to use purchased or prescribed medication form the major elements of the 'extended role'. These are largely encompassed within the *Pharmacy in a New Age: The New Horizon* document (Royal Pharmaceutical Society of Great Britain, 1996) which sees pharmacists, in the future, having greater involvement in the management of prescribed medicines and common ailments.

1. Advise patients on minor ailments
2. Advise patients on sensible and effective ways of using medicines
3. Provision of domiciliary services to housebound/isolated patients
4. Participation in continuing education of community health care practitioners
5. Health education and health promotion
6. Supervision of supply and safekeeping of medicines in residential and nursing homes
7. Keep records of prescribed and purchased medication
8. Registration of elderly patients
9. Advise prescribers on economic and effective prescribing and on the effects of medicines
10. Monitoring and reporting adverse drug reactions and interactions
11. Advising general practitioners on the administration and handling of complex substances
12. Diagnostic testing, e.g. measurement of blood pressure, blood glucose and cholesterol levels

Box 2.4 The pharmacist's 'extended role'

Studies of the British public's health have indicated that 91 per cent of individuals suffer from at least one minor ailment within a two-week period (British Market Research Bureau, 1997). Pharmacists in the community are uniquely placed to advise patients on the most appropriate and effective way of dealing with such ailments. Pharmacies are visited daily by an estimated 6 million people (Pharmaceutical Journal, 1988), including those who are healthy as well as those who are ill. Pharmacists are unique amongst health professionals in that they are readily available to the public, and can be consulted without the necessity of a prior appointment. They are therefore able both to advise on matters of health care (including lifestyle, nutrition etc.) and to provide treatment when necessary. Health care advice may be provided by the pharmacist through personal consultation and/or by the provision of educational literature. This aspect of the pharmacists' activities is discussed further in Chapter 8. Nevertheless, it should be noted that however enthusiastically pharmacists embrace the 'advice-giving' activities outlined in the extended role, the public still needs convincing that they have a need for such advice. A survey of 2,000 individuals revealed that a pharmacist's advice was sought in relation to only 1 per cent of the minor ailments they had experienced (British Market Research Bureau, 1997). This is in spite of extensive media advertising of pharmacists' availability and ability to give good advice, and an acceptance by the majority of adults that pharmacists are *a good source of advice/information about minor medical problems*' (British Market Research Bureau, 1997).

Other aspects of the 'extended role' depend on the pharmacist having a more active input into the delivery of primary health care. Pharmacists are participating more directly in the education of community health workers, such as those in residential homes for children, the handicapped and the elderly. Moreover, they are increasingly encouraged to assist in the supervision of the supply and safe keeping of the medicines in these institutions. Pharmacists may serve as a bridge between prescribers and community health workers, thereby enhancing the care of people in these establishments. Pharmacists now routinely keep medication records, allowing them to monitor the medication of their clients accurately and enabling them to identify potential drug interactions or contraindications for prescribed and purchased medication rapidly.

The ability of pharmacists to contribute to the control of prescribing costs is increasingly being recognised, such that they may now be employed within general practices to advise on cost-effective prescribing. A study of eight general practices in one health authority in England indicated that employing pharmacists was a cost-effective way of controlling prescribing expenditure, with considerable savings being made over and above the costs of employing the pharmacist (Rodgers *et al.*, 1999).

Much of what is encompassed in the extended role, together with pharmacists' traditional activities in relation to medicines supply, is captured by the terms 'pharmaceutical care' and 'medicines management'. Pharmaceutical care has been defined as '*the responsible provision of drug therapy for the purpose of achieving definite outcomes that improve a patient's quality of life*' (Hepler and Strand, 1990). Pharmaceutical care requires pharmacists to be directly responsible and accountable to patients for the outcomes of drug therapy, and as such presents the opportunity for pharmacists to manage medicines use. This correlates with medicines management, which is defined as '*the systematic provision of medicines therapy, through a partnership of effort between patients and professionals, to deliver best patient outcome at minimised cost*' (Tweedie, 2002).

Changes in the way pharmacists work is now inevitable. The UK government is seeking to optimise the use of pharmacists within the NHS and has recently stated that:

'*We wish to encourage . . . continued extension of the role of pharmacists in supporting patients, for example through medicines management schemes, medication review, local pharmaceutical services and other initiatives*' (Department of Health, 2002).

Pharmacist prescribing

In 1999, *A Review of the Prescribing, Supply and Administration of Medicines* (Crown, 1999) was published. Known as the Crown Report, among its recommendations was that some health professionals, other than doctors, should become either 'independent' or 'dependent' prescribers. Independent prescribers will be responsible for the initial assessment of patients, will devise the treatment plan, and will have the authority to prescribe the medicines required as part of that plan. Dependent prescribers will be authorised to prescribe certain medicines for patients whose condition has been previously diagnosed or assessed by an independent prescriber, within an agreed assessment and treatment plan. The government expects 1,000 pharmacists to be trained and prescribing by the end of 2004 (Pharmaceutical Journal, 2003) 'Pharmacist'/'supplementary' prescribing is a major initiative currently confronting the pharmacy profession. Whether pharmacists are ready, willing and capable of taking on such a function has yet to be properly established.

Currently, how the pharmaceutical profession can best fully implement the 'extended role' and prepare themselves for new activities, including prescribing, is still being debated. Persuading pharmacists to undertake new roles when they are predominantly paid, as a result of their contract with the NHS, for the supply of medicines and appliances against a prescriber's prescription is understandably problematic. Likewise, when pharmacists have become accustomed, and indeed required, to be personally involved in each dispensed prescription, often providing a 'final check', it is not surprising if they are resistant to attempts to relax the rules governing supervision by pharmacists in order to free up to perform additional (largely non-remunerated) functions. When immediately post-Nuffield the Royal Pharmaceutical Society proposed such a change an acrimonious debate within the pharmacy profession ensued, culminating in a special general meeting of the Royal Pharmaceutical Society of Great Britain in which a motion opposing the Society's council's proposals for such a relaxation was passed (Royal Pharmaceutical Society, 1989). In response to the government's proposals for change in health service delivery, published as the *NHS Plan* in 2000 (Department of Health, 2000b, 2000c), proposals to modify the supervision of dispensing by pharmacists requirements have again surfaced, and it seems likely that the detailed supervision of dispensing by pharmacists will be modified in the near future.

What is clear is that alongside changes in health care delivery in general, the role of the pharmacist has changed considerably in recent years, and will continue to change. As pharmacists become increasingly involved in new activities and have a greater input into primary and secondary health care, they have to acquire new knowledge and develop new skills if their input is to be significant, and if they are to remain at all credible in the eyes of other health professionals, to their paymasters (the State) and to the consumer of their services (the public).

SUMMARY

- More pharmacists practice in the community than in hospital
- Pharmacists' activities have traditionally centred around the dispensing of prescribed medication
- Pharmacists face new opportunities for developing their role
- Pharmacy is in a state of flux
- Pharmacists need to acquire and develop the appropriate skills if they are to effectively undertake proposed new activities, such as prescribing.

FURTHER READING

Hassell, K. and Symonds, S. (2001) The pharmacy workforce. In: K.M.G. Taylor and G. Harding (eds) *Pharmacy Practice*, London, Taylor and Francis, pp. 31–47.

Jesson, J. and Wilson, K. (1999) Primary care pharmacists: a conceptual model. *Pharmaceutical Journal*, 263, 62–64.

Stone, P. and Curtis, S.J. (2002) *Pharmacy Practice* (3rd edn), London, Pharmaceutical Press.

REFERENCES

Applebe, G.E. and Wingfield, J. (2001) *Dale and Applebe's Pharmacy Law and Ethics*, London, Pharmaceutical Press.

Audit Commission (2001) *A Spoonful of Sugar – Medicines Management in NHS Hospitals*, London, Audit Commision.

British Market Research Bureau Ltd (1997) *Everyday Healthcare Study of Self-medication in Great Britain*, London, The Proprietary Association of Great Britain.

Brookes, K., Scott, M.G. and McConnell, J.B. (2000) The benefits of a hospital based community services liaison pharmacist. *Pharmacy World Science*, 22, 33–38.

Crown, J. (1999) *A Review of the Prescribing, Supply and Administration of Medicines*, London, Department of Health.

Dean, B., Schachter, M., Vincent, C. and Barber, N. (2002) Prescribing errors in hospital inpatients – their incidence and clinical significance. *Quality and Safety in Health Care*, 11, 340–344.

Department of Health (2000a) *Statistical Bulletin 2000/20: Prescriptions Dispensed in the Community, Statistics for 1989 to 1999: England*, London, Department of Health.

Department of Health (2000b) *Pharmacy in the Future – Implementing the NHS Plan*, London, Department of Health.

Department of Health (2000c) *The NHS Plan: A Plan for Investment. A Plan for Reform*, London, The Stationery Office.

Department of Health (2002) *Pharmacy Workforce in the New NHS*, London, Department of Health.

DHSS (1986) *Primary Health Care: An Agenda for Discussion*, London, HMSO.

DHSS (1988) *Promoting Better Health*, London, HMSO.

Harding, G. and Taylor, K.M.G. (2000) The McDonaldisation of pharmacy. *Pharmaceutical Journal*, 265, 602.

Hassell, K. and Symonds, S. (2001) The pharmacy workforce. In: K.M.G. Taylor and G. Harding (eds) *Pharmacy Practice*, London, Taylor and Francis, pp. 31–47.

Hassell, K., Noyce, P. and Jesson, J. (1998) White and ethnic minority self-employment in retail pharmacy in Britain: an historical and comparative analysis. *Work, Employment and Society*, 12, 245–271.

Hassell, K., Fisher, R., Nichols, L. and Shann, P. (2002)

Contemporary workforce patterns and historical trends: the pharmacy labour market over the past 40 years. *Pharmaceutical Journal*, 269, 291–296.

Hepler, C.D. and Strand, L.M. (1990) Opportunities and responsibilities in pharmaceutical care. *American Journal of Hospital Pharmacy*, 47, 533–543.

Jesson, J. and Wilson, K. (1999) Primary care pharmacists: a conceptual model. *Pharmaceutical Journal*, 263, 62–64.

Jones, D.R. (1978) Errors on doctors' prescriptions. *Journal of the Royal College of General Practitioners*, 28, 543–545.

Neville, R.G., Robertson, F., Livingston, S. and Crombie, I.K. (1989) A classification of prescription errors. *Journal of the Royal College of General Practitioners*, 39, 110–112.

Nuffield Committee of Inquiry into Pharmacy (1986) *Pharmacy: A Report to the Nuffield Foundation*, London, Nuffield Foundation.

Pharmaceutical Journal (1988) Six million chances daily for health education. *Pharmaceutical Journal*, 241, 179.

Pharmaceutical Journal (1989) Pharmacist liable for doctor's error. *Pharmaceutical Journal*, 243, 186.

Pharmaceutical Journal (2001) Pharmacy numbers continue to fall slowly. *Pharmaceutical Journal*, 267, 875.

Pharmaceutical Journal (2003) Establishing training for pharmacist prescribing will be a challenge for 2003. *Pharmaceutical Journal*, 220, 7–8.

Ritzer, G. (2000) *The McDonaldization of Society* (2nd edn), Thousand Oaks, Calif., Pine Forge Press.

Rodgers, S., Avery, A.J. and Meechan, D. (1999) Controlled trial of pharmacist intervention in general practice: the effect on prescribing costs. *British Journal of General Practice*, 49, 717–720.

Royal Pharmaceutical Society of Great Britain (1989) Narrow but clear majority for no confidence motion. *Pharmaceutical Journal*, 242, 438.

Royal Pharmaceutical Society of Great Britain (1996) *Pharmacy in a New Age: The New Horizon*, London, The Royal Pharmaceutical Society of Great Britain.

Rutter, P.M., Hunt, A.J., Darracott, R. and Jones, I.F. (1998) A subjective study of how community pharmacists in Great Britain Spend their time. *Journal of Social and Administrative Pharmacy*, 15, 252–261.

Shah, S.N., Aslam, M. and Avery, A.J. (2001) A survey of prescription errors in general practice. *Pharmaceutical Journal*, 267, 860–863.

Tweedie, A. (2002) Medicines management and change management – the PSNC pilot trials. *Pharmaceutical Journal*, 268, 146.

Zermansky, A.G., Petty, D.R., Raynor, D.K., Freemantle, N., Vail, A. and Lowe, C.J. (2001) Randomised controlled trial of clinical medication review by a pharmacist of elderly patients receiving repeat prescriptions in general practice. *British Medical Journal*, 323, 1340–1343.

INTRODUCTION

In this chapter we examine the ways in which individuals experience and exhibit symptoms of illness, and explore the factors that influence their responses to those symptoms. The chapter illustrates that the experience of symptoms does not inevitably result in people seeking help from a health professional. Rather, the way in which people respond to symptoms is more complex than might at first be imagined. For instance, it may be assumed that a simple correlation exists between the severity of symptoms and the decision to consult a health professional. In other words, we might predict that the worse an individual feels the more likely they are to seek professional health care. In reality, the utilisation of health services is influenced by a wide range of factors which sometimes override the severity of the symptoms. Many of these factors have been identified and studied since the inception of the National Health Service in 1948.

Much of the thinking behind the policies which led to the foundation of the National Health Service in the 1940s rested on the premise that people who experience symptoms or ill-health would seek medical aid if the services were readily available and free at the point of use. Moreover, it was believed that after the creation of a universally free service there would be a dramatic rise in the demand for medical care, but that once the backlog of ill-health in the community had been treated, this demand would stabilise, and the need and demand for such services would, in time, become more stable. However, the reality did not match this apparent logic. This was due to a lack of awareness and understanding about the nature and prevalence of illness symptoms in the community, and of how people interpret and make sense of their experiences of health and illness.

ILLNESS AS A SOCIAL CONCEPT

In order to understand how patients respond to ill-health it is useful to appreciate the differences between illness and disease. Disease refers to a pathological or biological condition, for example cancer of the lung or kidney failure. Illness, on the other hand, concerns individuals' responses to symptoms: how they feel, experience and make sense of their sickness. Illness and disease are not therefore synonymous – it is possible to feel ill without suffering a disease and to suffer a disease without feeling ill. For instance, a woman who has cervical cancer may feel perfectly healthy, whilst someone who is ill through excessive stress may not exhibit a pathological disease. The distinction between illness and disease is important because it emphasises the fact that the way in which people respond to symptoms is often as important as the disease state itself. However, this distinction can be misleading because disease itself is not unequivocal. Pathological norms have changed over time and are not universally accepted. Comparative studies indicate that what counts as disease in one setting may be considered normal in another (McElroy and Jezewski, 2000).

The boundary between sickness and health is not clear-cut. Illness is a variance from normality, and what is 'normal' varies between societies, cultures, and groups within society. In this sense illness is a socially defined concept – that is, the implicit meaning of illness is not universally shared but is peculiar to specific cultures and societies.

Illness behaviour

The presence of symptoms alone does not determine the use of health services. Instead, uptake of these services is to a large extent determined by how individuals respond to these symptoms. The study of 'illness behaviour' is the study of behaviour in its social context, rather than in relation to a physiological or pathological condition. Being sick can be regarded as an active process, not a passive state; that is to say, to be ill involves the individual (and others) in making interpretations about their symptoms, making a choice of what to do about their experience of illness or sickness, and finally deciding what course of action to take in response to the symptoms – to attempt to alleviate them or to simply ignore them. Illness behaviour, then, is a sociological concept which attempts to describe how people respond to their symptoms. This implies that the way in which symptoms are perceived, evaluated and acted upon is influenced by people's previous health-related experiences and an individual's social environment.

There are two perspectives on illness behaviour which have been identified and termed as 'individualistic' and 'collectivist' approaches (Morgan *et al.*, 1985). Individualistic approaches stress the characteristics of the individual, whilst the collectivist approaches emphasise the shared social norms and values that influence the actions of people within social groups.

Ten variables have been identified which may influence an individual's response to illness (Box 3.1). These factors are undoubtedly relevant considerations which influence an individual's response to illness. However, collectivist approaches point out that illness behaviour is a culturally learned response; in other words, the experience of illness is defined according to the prevailing norms and values of a society or community. It is not the symptoms themselves that are significant in comprehending illness behaviour, but the way in which the symptoms are defined and interpreted. Symptoms which are considered to be normal in one context may be considered to be abnormal in another.

	1. Visibility, recognisability or perceived importance of deviant signs and symptoms 2. The extent to which a person's symptoms are perceived as serious; that is, the person's estimate of the present and future probabilities of danger indicated by these symptoms 3. The extent to which symptoms disrupt family life, work and other social activities 4. The frequency of the appearance of the deviant signs and symptoms, their persistence, or the frequency of their recurrence 5. The tolerance threshold of those who are exposed to and evaluate the deviant signs and symptoms 6. Available information, knowledge and cultural assumptions and understandings of the evaluator 7. Psychological factors that lead to denial of symptoms – for example, fear of confirmation of disease, such as cancer 8. More pressing or immediate needs may compete with illness responses – for example, work commitments may be regarded as more important than dealing with illness 9. Competing possible interpretations that can be assigned to the symptoms once they are recognised 10. Availability of treatment resources, physical proximity, and psychological and monetary costs of taking action. Included are not only physical distance and costs of time, money and effort, but also costs such as social stigma, social distance and feelings of humiliation

Box 3.1 Variables which may influence response to illness (Mechanic, 1968)

This 'normalising' process is a common and frequent part of everyday life. However, when symptoms prevent a person from behaving 'normally', as expected by themselves or others, then the symptoms may no longer be considered 'normal'. In this event, a search for explanations to make sense of the symptom may ensue. For example, whether two individuals with a persistent cough experience this symptom in the same way will depend on a number of social factors. A person living in a damp house may interpret their early morning hacking cough as 'normal', not as something out of the ordinary, an everyday experience shared by neighbours which does not require presentation to a health care professional. A person with a similar cough living in a centrally heated house might perceive this symptom quite differently – as a sign of possible serious illness requiring urgent professional health care. We can see, then, that people evaluate their physical and/or emotional sensations in terms of their existing knowledge, experience and advice from other people. Hence, when we talk of illness behaviour we are saying that responses to symptoms are learned in accordance with the individual's social environment.

Within any social environment there may be different cultures. Cultural differences may be significant in determining how individuals interpret and respond to their symptoms. However, it has also been pointed out that it is possible to identify responses to illness which are common to groups of individuals. For example, in a study of North Americans of Irish and Italian descent, a direct link between the membership of a cultural group and the communication of bodily complaints was established. Their response to illness reflected that of their responses to their other troubles and problems. The Irish-Americans responded to their symptoms by denial of their sickness, whilst the Italians responded by dramatisation (Zola, 1966). A similar study conducted in New York in the 1950s (Zborowski, 1952) found that patients of Old-American or Irish origin displayed a pragmatic attitude towards pain and, when it was particularly intense, they showed a tendency to withdraw from the company of others. By contrast, individuals of Italian or Jewish background tended to be more demanding and dependent as patients and were inclined to seek sympathy. Of course we must be cautious here, these findings reveal that responses to symptoms are contingent upon not only the social milieu in which people reside but also their historical context, and so if the study were to be replicated today it is likely that the findings may well be different.

Morgan and Watkins (1988) have explored the perceptions and responses of sixty-two European 'white' and West Indian patients with hypertension. Although both groups of patients were aware of the importance of controlling their blood pressure, and all identified stress as a causal factor, they differed in their attitude to antihypertensive medication. Almost all (twenty-six out of thirty) of the 'white' respondents said they took the medications as prescribed, compared with only twelve of the thirty West Indian respondents. The 'leaving off' of medication by the West Indian patients was explained by their concern about the long-term adverse effects of drug use, and their dislike of being dependent on medicines. Some of these patients also questioned the need to take drugs if they felt all right. Moreover, the partial rejection of long-term drug therapy by this group was associated with the use of herbal remedies taken as well as, or as an alternative to, their prescribed medication. More recently, Benson and Britten (2002) have shown choices regarding the taking of antihypertensive medicines involved patients in weighing up their reservations of taking medication against the perceived positive benefits of doing so. The authors recommended that doctors who wanted their patients to make well-informed choices about antihypertensive medication should explore how individuals strike this balance between reservations about and reasons for taking their medicines.

How people make sense of, and respond to their symptoms can in some circumstances be a matter of life or death. For example, one study on help-seeking for myocardial infarction found that 40 per cent of patients who experienced symptoms delayed calling for help for more than four hours (Leslie *et al.*, 2000). A qualitative study that examined hospital patients' treatment decisions reveals some of the reasons for delay (Clark, 2001). Symptoms, typically chest pain, were sometimes thought to be 'familiar' and it was only when they became significantly more severe that they were perceived as being perhaps out of the ordinary. Furthermore, symptoms were thought to be symptomatic of benign illness, for which people employed 'tried and tested' strategies, such as taking an oral medication or getting rest and sleep. In sum, as we have discussed above, people routinely tend to normalise symptoms and it is only when they appear very out of the ordinary that they consider seeking emergency help.

Frequency of symptoms: the symptom iceberg

Today, we realise that the majority of symptoms experienced by people are not presented to a health professional. Most people either fail to perceive their symptoms, or ignore, tolerate or self-treat them. The fact that the majority of symptoms are not presented to a health professional has been referred to by Hannay (1979) as the *'symptom iceberg'*. This is represented diagrammatically in Figure 3.1.

Surveys of the general population have shown that symptoms are frequently experienced by most adults. Evidence of the frequent experience of symptoms was reported in a study of women aged 16–44 years (Scambler *et al.*, 1981). These women were asked to keep a diary of any occurrence of illness. Symptoms were recorded on average one day in three, but only one medical consultation was sought for every eighteen recorded symptoms.

Further evidence of the frequent experience of symptoms was found in a study of the incidence of illness amongst 2,000 adults in

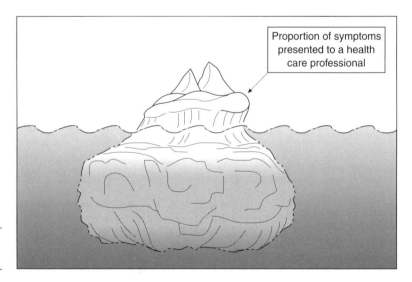

Proportion of symptoms presented to a health care professional

Figure 3.1 The symptom iceberg

Illness	Adults reporting illness in previous two weeks (%)
Tiredness	40
Headache	33
Muscle aches or pains	29
Sleeping problems	23
Stiffness in joints	22
Back problems	20
Bruising	17
Stress or anxiety	17
Feeling low or depressed	16
Minor cuts and grazes	16
Common cold	14
Arthritis	14
Acne	12
Hangover	12

Table 3.1 Incidence of reported illness over a two-week period (reproduced with permission from British Market Research Bureau, 1997)

Great Britain (British Market Research Bureau, 1997). This study found that 91 per cent of the individuals interviewed reported experiencing at least one ailment during the previous two weeks (Table 3.1) with an average of 5.2 ailments in a two-week period. These ailments included some which were acute, some which were chronic and others which were recurrent in nature.

In response to these ailments 46 per cent of those interviewed took no action at all. Thirty-four per cent used an over the counter (OTC) medicine or home remedy, whilst only 10 per cent saw a doctor or dentist and 1 per cent sought the advice of a pharmacist (Table 3.2).

Thus, whilst the range and incidence of symptoms in the population as a whole has been found to be very high the proportion of people who actively seek professional help in response to these symptoms is low. These findings correspond well with those of earlier studies. For instance, Wadsworth *et al.* (1971), in a study of the incidence of symptoms over two weeks in two London boroughs, found that of 1,000 randomly selected individuals, 19 per cent experienced symptoms but took no action, 56 per cent who experienced symptoms took some form of self-medication, 17 per cent consulted with a general practitioner, whilst 3 per cent were

Table 3.2 The response of adults to minor ailments (reproduced with permission from British Market Research Bureau, 1997)

Response	Percentage
Did not use anything	46
Used a prescription medicine already in the house	14
Used an OTC medicine	25
Used a 'home remedy' (e.g. hot-water bottle)	9
Saw a doctor or dentist	10
Saw a pharmacist	1

outpatients and 0.5 per cent were inpatients in hospital. Only 5 per cent reported experiencing no symptoms at all.

Not only does the presence of a symptom not necessarily precipitate a consultation with a health professional, but there is also evidence that decisions of whether or not to visit a health professional do not simply depend on the severity of the symptom itself. For example, it has been found that patients who suffered from severe facial pain did not seek professional treatment (Marbach and Lipton, 1978).

The existence of a 'symptom iceberg' has significant implications for health care in general and pharmaceutical service delivery in particular. These studies have revealed that there is a reservoir of untreated minor symptoms and ailments within the community, some, if not most, of which could be dealt with effectively by the pharmacist. Seemingly 'minor' ailments could be evaluated by the pharmacist as to whether or not they are self-limiting, treatable with an OTC medicine or warrant the attention of, for example, a general practitioner, a specialist clinic, a dentist or a chiropodist.

The worried well

In contrast to the majority of the population who on experiencing minor ailments will either self-medicate or do nothing, a number of developments in recent years have given rise to the concept of the 'worried well'. These are individuals who recognise their potential for illness and unnecessarily seek reassurance, or confirmatory tests from health care providers (Fitzpatrick, 2001). Healthy patients who regard minor aches and pains with considerable foreboding have always existed. However, the increase in this behaviour reflects technological advances, changes in the relationships between users and providers of health care, and not least the increasing perception of 'risk' in individuals' lives. Technological developments in screening for diseases, the introduction of highly effective pharmaceuticals, the open accessibility of medical knowledge via the media and over the World Wide Web, and not least the Human Genome Project, have created a capacity for people who are increasingly aware of their potential for illness to seek health care, often inappropriately. Anxieties about health are compounded by 'health scares' which are becoming more frequent. Health issues such as the risks associated with the combined mumps, measles and rubella (MMR) vaccine, genetically modified food and variant CJD – the human form of mad cow disease/BSE – are examples of such 'scares'.

THE EXPERIENCE OF CHRONIC ILLNESS

In post-industrial societies chronic illnesses are more prevalent than infectious and acute conditions. The major illnesses that affect people today include cancers, heart disease, asthma and diabetes. Chronic illnesses are, by definition, incurable and so this means that sufferers have to learn how to live with and manage their conditions. The management of illness involves striking a balance between medical imperatives, such as drug treatments and therapies, and social considerations such as adapting one's social life. Because people have to learn to live with their symptoms they may soon become experts in the management of them. Indeed, this has been recognised by governments in both the UK and North America in the so-called 'expert patient' initiative whereby patients are supported through the care of their own health (see Chapter 4).

Sociological studies of chronic illness have identified a number of themes which appear to be relevant to a wide range of conditions. These relate to the management of chronic illness, coping strategies, stigma and the impact that illness may have on an individual's sense of self and identity. It is evident from this research that the biophysical changes may have significant social consequences. Chronic illness may impact upon a person's daily living, their social relationships, their social identity (the view others hold of them) and their sense of self (their private view of themselves). Thus illness is at once both a very personal and a very public phenomenon.

Strategies that people pursue to manage their illness involve actions that are common to all of us. These might include weighing up the pros and cons of taking certain actions, making choices and decisions about how best to accomplish tasks and to achieve goals. A sociological study into people's experiences of Parkinson's Disease found that these processes of 'balancing' became more intensified and more precarious in the face of an illness which is characterised by uncertainty and unpredictability (Pinder, 1988). For example, sufferers often have to weigh up the costs and benefits of taking drugs which might both alleviate symptoms and result in unpleasant adverse effects. It is difficult to assess the balance in the face of uncertainty about the possible onset of symptoms themselves which often come and go without any apparent reason. There are also decisions to be made about carrying on as normal and not telling others about one's illness and risking the possibility that it may become evident. This has to be balanced against the consequences of disclosing to others that one has a particular condition, or avoiding situations where people might find out, which may in turn result in stigma and potential social isolation (Nijhof, 2002).

The experience of chronic illness can very often mean a severe reduction in resources in terms of energy, skill, strength, time, money, friends, and so on. As a result sufferers adopt strategies to overcome these restrictions. Corbin and Strauss (1985) have usefully observed that such strategies can be conceptualised as forms of 'work'. They further propose that responses to chronic illness can be understood in terms of various types of work. First, 'illness work', which consists of regimen work (e.g. taking drugs, applying therapies), crisis prevention and management, symptom management and diagnostic related work. Second, relatedly, there is 'information work' which involves networking, seeking out information and advice about a condition and treatments, and searching for types of health care provision. This may involve anything from gathering leaflets, contacting health care providers for information, and trawling the Internet for advice, information and support. Third, 'everyday life work' refers to the daily round of tasks that keep a household going, such as housekeeping, occupational work, child rearing, sentimental work and activities such as preparing and eating food. Fourth, 'biographical work' which involves the reconstruction of the ill person's biography.

Sociologists have suggested that the onset of chronic illness can be understood as a 'biographical disruption' (Bury, 1982) in that it can disturb not only one's physical body but also one's whole life on a number of levels. As Bury (1982) explains:

'First, there is the disruption of taken-for-granted assumptions and behaviours. Second, there are more profound disruptions in explanatory systems normally used by people such that a fundamental rethinking of a person's biography and self concept is involved. Third, there is a response to disruption involving the mobilization of resources in facing an altered situation.'

The impact of a chronic condition will of course vary according to the nature and severity of the illness, and also when the onset of the condition occurred. Although chronic illness can profoundly alter people's lives, research has also revealed how people are well able to accommodate and normalise their experiences.

For example, a study which examined the lives of children who had been diagnosed with asthma found that both parents and children tended to 'downplay' their symptoms (Prout *et al.*, 1999). The authors of this study argue that this is important because the bulk of medical research into the social outcomes of asthma has focused upon the negative aspects of the condition. They propose an 'adaptive perspective', which they argue must pay attention to the changing experiences of the sufferer and recognise how successful strategies for coping can contribute to a sense of achievement and esteem for the sufferer. This 'adaptive perspective' is implicit in the work of Williams (2000) who analysed children's accounts of living with both diabetes and asthma. She noted that responses to illness were gendered – in other words, boys and girls tended to respond differently to their diseases. Whilst boys were keen to downplay their illness and associated symptoms, girls did not. Girls were more likely than boys to tell others about their illness, use their medication in public settings and were more likely to incorporate their conditions into their social identities. Boys were not keen to incorporate the illness into their personal and social identities. However, there was a small minority of boys who felt that although they had been able to control their symptoms in the past and so 'pass as normal', they no longer could do so. This had made them feel angry about their illness and they felt it led to their identities being 'denigrated' (Williams, 2000).

LAY KNOWLEDGE AND BELIEFS ABOUT ILLNESS AND HEALTH

The biographical quality of people's views was identified and developed by Williams and Wood (1986) in their research of people who suffered from arthritis. They revealed that patients have a genuine and urgent interest in understanding why they have the disease, and develop 'models' in order to explain and make sense of it. The sufferers also had additional purposes which played an important part in determining the choice of their beliefs; these included the need to locate etiological explanations within their own life experiences.

An example quoted by Williams and Wood (1986) was of a man who explained the cause of his rheumatoid arthritis as being a direct result of specific life experiences, which included stress incurred during the war when he had worked in a bomb disposal unit, and also his long-term exposure to the natural elements when he was employed on a building site. These events were regarded by the sufferer to be important contributory factors to his disease; but it was after a post-operative infection that he felt his arthritis had really *'gone to town'*.

Similarly, in a study of views about disease, Blaxter (1983) found that the forty-six women interviewed developed causal models to explain their bouts of illness, which displayed a high degree of sophistication. Social factors were recognised as mediating between an ultimate cause and the onset of illness. For example, influenza was believed to be caused by a virus, but factors such as general susceptibility to such an illness, being run down and getting wet, as when for example being caught in a storm, all entered into their explanations. Thus, whilst these women acknowledged the bio-medical cause of the illness, this was interpreted in the light of their life experiences.

Lay health beliefs

As we have seen, people's responses to symptoms are many, varied and diverse. Ideas and beliefs about health are derived from many sources and have also been the subject of study by medical sociologists. The first sociological studies of people's views of health and illness appeared in the early 1960s (Apple, 1960; Freidson, 1961). This interest in what people think and have to say about health and illness has resulted in a variety of studies in which their ideas and beliefs have been defined and analysed. The ideas of individuals with regard to health and illness are referred to in the sociological literature as 'lay health beliefs'. An understanding of lay health beliefs is useful and important because it serves to:

1. Enhance our understanding of the social impact and meaning of health, disease and illness.
2. Enhance the health professional–patient relationship.
3. Allow the development of realistic approaches and strategies in health education and promotion.
4. Allow the development of appropriate health services based on the perceived needs of sufferers rather than on the perceptions of health care providers.

Using qualitative research methods (described in Chapter 9), a number of sociologists have researched the form and content of lay beliefs about health and illness in Western communities. A significant finding from this work is the confirmation that lay ideas concerning health are not simply crude distortions of medical knowledge but that they often display their own logic, coherence and sophistication. Indeed, as we have already seen, lay accounts have an experiential or biographical quality. Furthermore, an individual may hold a multiplicity of ideas about disease and illness, drawing from a range of information sources which include both formal medical knowledge and informal belief systems. This is as true for health professionals as it is for non-professionals. For example, a study of general practitioners in North London found that these doctors concurrently articulated ideas about colds and flu that made use of both clinical and popular knowledge, and what is more they prescribed treatments and care on the basis of such knowledge (Helman, 1978).

Multiplicity of ideas model

In a study of patients' beliefs about hypertension, Blumhagen (1980) found ten different kinds of causal factors which were commonly cited by sufferers. These included chronic external stress, genetic make up, and salt and water intake. Blumhagen further found that some respondents gave unrelated explanations for the cause of their hypertension at different stages of the interview. It is of interest to note that when confronted by these differing explanations, the patients did not feel that this presented problems or was in any way inconsistent. Each explanation was derived from a different source and within its context made sense. To describe this quality of lay health beliefs, Fitzpatrick *et al.* (1984) have referred to them as 'syncretic', by which they mean *'ideas are drawn selectively from a variety of different traditions and adjusted according to the current concerns of the individual'*.

Comparative studies of lay beliefs about the aetiology of illness have helped us to appreciate that people's ideas and beliefs, which may at first appear strange, do contain their own rationale and logic. It is evident that the search for an explanation of the cause of illness is important to people who experience that illness. Chrisman (1977), in a review of the literature from different cultures on lay ideas about the aetiology of disease, identified four commonly used explanations to account for the pathology of the body in the event of ill-health.

1. *Invasion*: the rationale that the body is susceptible to intrusion of matter or substances that are able to make the body ill, such as micro-organisms, toxic chemicals, or spoiled food.
2. *Degeneration*: whereby the body is perceived and expected to get progressively worse with age.
3. *Mechanical*: the structure or functioning of the body is impeded as the result of blockages, fractures, breakdowns, etc.
4. *Balance*: the imperative of maintaining an equilibrium between elements within the body and between the body and the environment.

People's health beliefs are particularly relevant in relation to so-called 'behavioural diseases' such as Acquired Immune Deficiency Syndrome (AIDS). In a study titled 'Constructing common sense – young people's beliefs about AIDS', Warwick *et al.* (1988) stress three reasons why young people's views are important:

1. Lay beliefs may temper the effectiveness of the official health education messages which rely on professional and bio-medical explanations to inform people about the causes of AIDS.
2. People's ideas and beliefs are likely to influence their perception of 'risks.'
3. Lay beliefs have an impact on the way disease is understood and interpreted, and thus experienced.

Models of lay health beliefs

It has been suggested that there must be a relationship between health beliefs and behaviour. Attempts to understand this relationship can be divided into socio-psychological approaches and sociological approaches. A characteristic of the former have been the attempts to construct models which can be used to explain and describe the impact that health beliefs have on health behaviours. One such model is the Health Belief Model (HBM) (Rosenstock, 1966; Becker, 1974). The HBM attempts to identify motives which influence people's health-related actions and tries to recognise those which are most vulnerable to change. Factors such as age and sex would be immutable; however, subjective factors in the form of people's perceptions would be alterable. The dimensions of the HBM are:

- the level of interest an individual expresses in health issues (health motivation)
- their perceived vulnerability to illness (susceptibility)
- the perceived seriousness of certain illnesses (severity)
- the perceived value of taking health actions (benefits and costs).

An assessment of these perceptions, it is argued, will enable the researcher or health educator to identify the likelihood and willingness of the individual to comply with 'desirable' health behaviours. This argument is particularly attractive to health educators because if it is possible to identify ways in which behaviour can be changed they could act upon and advise those who do not subscribe to healthy actions. However, social reality is not so straightforward. The HBM is therefore an individualistic interpretation because there is an assumption that if people have the appropriate motives and perceptions they will undertake professionally prescribed health routines and actions. As such, it underestimates the wider social constraints and circumstances in which people live. It also takes the value of professionally defined actions as a given and, as a corollary, underplays alternative non-professional, health-related actions.

Studies which have attempted to evaluate the HBM have found that the level of variance in behaviour as a function of health belief/motivational variables is small and thus the predictive value of the model is negligible (Calnan, 1984). This highlights as problematic a fundamental assumption on which the HBM is based – that is, to what extent can we assume a correlative relation between belief and behaviour or between knowledge, experience and action? This has important implications for health promotion and disease prevention, discussed in Chapter 8. We also expand upon these ideas in the following chapter when we explore the actions people take to seek help when they experience symptoms or illness.

SUMMARY

- It can be helpful to distinguish between disease and illness – the former refers to pathological or biological changes, the latter to how symptoms are experienced
- The concept of 'illness behaviour' reveals that responses to symptoms are shaped by the social, cultural and historical context in which an individual resides
- A 'symptom iceberg' exists, in that the vast majority of symptoms are not seen by health practitioners and the majority are either self-treated, ignored or simply tolerated
- Chronic illnesses are the most common in post-industrial societies and people who suffer from them develop considerable expertise in the management of their conditions
- Lay health knowledge is characterised by its complexity and sophistication and people are able to draw on a wide range of sometimes competing sources of information
- Before pharmacists are called upon to respond to symptoms they have already been 'interpreted' by the patient.

FURTHER READING

Bytheway, B., Johnson, J. and Heller, T. (2000) *The Management of Long Term Medication by Older People*, Milton Keynes, Open University Press.

Davey, B., Gray, A. and Seale, C. (eds) (2001) *Health and Disease; a Reader*, Buckingham, The Open University Press.

Nettleton, S. (1995) *The Sociology of Health and Illness*, Cambridge, Polity Press.

Nettleton, S. and Gustafsson, G. (eds) (2002) *The Sociology of Health and Illness Reader*, Cambridge, Polity Press.

White, K. (2002) *An Introduction to the Sociology of Health and Illness*, London, Sage.

REFERENCES

Apple, D. (1960) How laymen define illness. *Human Behaviour*, 1, 219–225.

Becker, M.H. (1974) *The Health Belief Model and Personal Health Behavior*. Thorofare, N.J., Charles B. Slack Inc.

Benson, J. and Britten, N. (2002) Patients' decisions about whether or not to take antihypertensive drugs: qualitative study. *British Medical Journal*, 325, 873–878.

Blaxter, M. (1983) The causes of disease: women talking. *Social Science and Medicine*, 17, 59–69.

Blumhagen, D. (1980) Hyper-tension: a folk illness with a medical name. *Culture, Medicine and Psychiatry*, 4, 197–227.

British Market Research Bureau Ltd (1997) *Everyday Healthcare Study of Self-medication in Great Britain*, London, The Proprietary Association of Great Britain.

Bury, M. (1982) Chronic illness as a biographical disruption. *Sociology of Health and Illness*, 4, 167–182.

Calnan, M. (1984) The Health Belief Model and participation programmes for the early detection of breast cancer: a comparative analysis. *Social Science and Medicine*, 19, 823–830.

Chrisman, N.J. (1977) The health seeking process: an approach to the natural history of illness. *Culture, Medicine and Society*, 1, 351–377.

Clark, A.M. (2001) Treatment decision-making during the early stages of heart attack: a case for the role of body and self in influencing delays. *Sociology of Health and Illness* 23, 425–447.

Corbin, J. and Strauss, A. (1985) Managing chronic illness at home: three lines of work. *Qualitative Sociology*, 8, 224–247.

Fitzpatrick, M. (2001) *The Tyranny of Health: Doctors and the Regulation of Lifestyle*, London, Routledge.

Fitzpatrick, R., Hinton, J., Newman, S., Scambler, G. and Thompson, J. (1984) *The Experience of Illness*, London, Tavistock.

Freidson, E. (1961) *Patients' Views of Medical Practice*, New York, Russell Sage Foundation.

Hannay, R. (1979) *The Symptom Iceberg: a Study in Community Health*, London, Routledge and Kegan Paul.

Helman, C. (1978) 'Feed a cold and starve a fever' – folk models of infection in an English suburban community and their relation to medical treatment. *Culture, Medicine and Psychiatry*, 2, 107–137.

Leslie, W.S., Urie, A., Hooper, J. and Morrison, C.E. (2000) Delay in calling for help during myocardial infarction: reasons for delay and subsequent patterns of accessing care. *Heart*, 84, 137–141.

Marbach, J.J. and Lipton, J.A. (1978) Aspects of illness behavior in patients with facial pain. *Journal of the American Dental Association*, 96, 630–638.

McElroy, A. and Jezewski, M.A. (2000) Cultural variation in the experience of health and illness. In: G.L. Albrecht, R. Fitzpatrick and S.C. Scrimshaw (eds) *The Handbook of Social Studies in Health and Medicine*, London, Sage, pp. 191–209.

Mechanic, D. (1968) *Medical Sociology: A Selective View*, New York, Free Press.

Morgan, M. and Watkins, C.J. (1988) Managing hypertension beliefs and responses to medication among cultural groups. *Sociology of Health and Illness*, 10, 561–578.

Morgan, M., Calnan, M. and Manning, N. (1985) *Sociological Approaches to Health and Medicine*, London, Routledge and Kegan Paul.

Nijhof, G. (2002) Parkinson's Disease as a problem of shame in public appearance. In: S. Nettleton and U. Gustafsson (eds) *The Sociology of Health and Illness Reader*, Cambridge, Polity Press, pp. 188–196.

Pinder, R. (1988) Striking balances: living with Parkinson's Disease. In: R. Anderson and M. Bury (eds) *Living with Chronic Illness: The Experience of Patients and their Families*, London, Unwin Hyman, pp. 67–88.

Prout, A., Hayes, L. and Gelder, L. (1999) Medicines and the maintenance of ordinariness in the household management of childhood asthma. *Sociology of Health and Illness*, 21, 137–162.

Rosenstock, I. (1966) Why people use health services. *Milbank Memorial Fund Quarterly*, 44, 94–127.

Scambler, A., Scambler, G. and Craig, D. (1981) Kinship and friendship networks and women's demands for primary care. *Journal of the Royal College of General Practitioners*, 26, 746–750.

Wadsworth, M., Butterfield, W. and Blaney, R. (1971) *Health and Sickness: The Choice of Treatment*, London, Tavistock Publications.

Warwick, I., Aggleton, P. and Homans, H. (1988) Constructing common sense – young people's beliefs about AIDS. *Sociology of Health and Illness*, 10, 213–233.

Williams, C. (2000) Doing health, doing gender: teenagers, diabetes and asthma. *Social Science and Medicine*, 50, 387–396.

Williams, G.H. and Wood, P.H.N. (1986) Common sense beliefs about illness: a mediating role for the doctor. *Lancet*, ii, 1435–1437.

Zborowski, M. (1952) Cultural components in response to pain. *Journal of Social Issues*, 8, 16–30.

Zola, I.K. (1966) Culture and symptoms, an analysis of patients presenting complaints. *American Sociological Review*, 31, 615–630.

4 Seeking Help and Consulting Health Professionals

INTRODUCTION

The promotion of pharmacists as a 'first port of call' for members of the public seeking advice on minor ailments or general health advice forms a cornerstone of strategies for pharmacists to extend their activities beyond those with which they are traditionally associated – namely, the dispensing of medicines and sale of medicines over the counter (see Chapters 2 and 7). Magazine, television and radio advertising has been employed to encourage the public to consult their pharmacist, as an 'expert', for health advice. However, as we have seen in Chapter 3, the decision-making process leading to people seeking professional health care or advice is not 'triggered' simply by the onset or the severity of symptoms. Rather, what is more significant is how the symptoms are perceived and interpreted. Furthermore, actions taken in response to symptoms are mediated by other factors such as the 'costs' and 'benefits' of seeking help, and the responses of friends, colleagues and relatives to an individual's illness. This chapter examines the social context of seeking help in response to illness. An understanding of this context is necessary prior to a discussion of interactions or 'consultations' between health care providers and their clients.

CONSULTATION AS A SOCIAL PROCESS

The pharmacist is ideally positioned to contribute substantially towards meeting the public's need for health care advice and treatment, particularly where existing services are inappropriate or inadequate. Many general practitioners complain that they are frequently consulted for what they consider to be 'trivial conditions'. Of 2,000 individuals interviewed about minor ailments and self-medication, 58 per cent said that they had consulted their general practitioner in the previous twelve months regarding minor or common ailments (British Market Research Bureau, 1997). Moreover, in one national study it was reported that a quarter of the general practitioners questioned felt that half or more of their surgery consultations fell into this category (Cartwright and Anderson, 1981). Many of these conditions which might be considered to be trivial by the general practitioner could be more suitably dealt with by community pharmacists. It is nevertheless important to appreciate that whilst complaints may be considered trivial by a general practitioner they may be very significant to the patient. Furthermore, as we discussed in the previous chapter, only a minority of symptoms are actually brought to the attention of a health practitioner.

Initiating a consultation with a health care professional

An individual's decision when or indeed whether or not to use health care services is influenced by their immediate network of family and friends, their values and beliefs and their attitudes towards professional health care. An American sociologist, Irving Zola, has established five types of responses whereby a symptom may be experienced by a patient as being abnormal, thereby triggering the individual to seek health care advice. Zola (1973) identified these triggers as:

1. *Perceived interference with vocational or physical activity*. If the experience of a symptom or symptoms begins to interfere with an individual's routine ability to work or to take part in routine physical activity, then the symptom(s) may be regarded as 'abnormal'.

2. *Perceived interference with social or personal relations*. Cause for concern may arise when the experience of symptoms interferes with one's normal patterns of social interaction. Of course what is considered normal will differ from individual to individual, depending on such factors as occupation, lifestyle, age, and so forth.

3. *The occurrence of an interpersonal crisis*. During periods of stable and harmonious interpersonal relationships, common and trivial symptoms may be regarded as inoffensive. The breakdown of such relationships can however, have profound effects on the way symptoms are experienced. Symptoms that were previously barely perceived, might, in the course of an interpersonal crisis, suddenly be discerned as a threat to health. Interpersonal crises can also diminish people's ability to cope with long-standing symptoms. Strategies for coping with a chronic pain can be undermined by interpersonal crises, and result in an enhanced perception of that pain.

4. *Temporalising symptoms*. Another trigger may be the persistence of a symptom, which may or may not interfere with work or personal relations, though nonetheless remaining a source of concern or puzzlement to the particular individual. This may lead the person to decide to give the symptom a set number of days or weeks to abate. In the event of the symptom not improving during this time, then the individual may seek professional help. This is exemplified by statements such as *'if it's not better by Monday I'll do something about it'*.

5. *Sanctioning*. While the person experiencing the symptoms may feel they do not warrant professional attention, perceiving them instead as either trivial or unimportant, pressure exerted by family or friends may lead them to visit a health professional. Similarly, the symptom may be a cause of anxiety to the sufferer but they may choose to avoid seeking professional help

for fear that their complaint may be considered trivial. Confirmation from family or friends that they have a legitimate claim for professional help may trigger the sufferer to take appropriate action.

We can see from Zola's triggers that it is not simply a question of being, or not being, conscious of symptoms, nor their severity, which necessarily determines what is to be done about them. The role of friends, families and colleagues is also a major factor in this process.

LAY REFERRAL SYSTEMS

The decision to act upon symptoms is not necessarily taken exclusively by the sufferer, but is often the result of discussions with a range of people – either immediate members of an individual's family, their friends or colleagues. Freidson (1970) refers to this network of friends, relatives and colleagues as the 'lay referral system'. The decision to use or avoid professional health care services, Freidson maintains, is influenced by:

- the extent of 'close knit social relations' between the members who make up a person's lay referral system, and
- the predominant values and attitudes to professional health care within that lay referral system.

For example, whether or not a person lives in an extended family (i.e. where people have daily or frequent contact with a range of relatives such as parents, grandparents, aunts and uncles), or the extent to which their ideas of health and illness do, or do not, match those of health professionals, or whether or not people live relatively independent of others, may each play a part in influencing an individual's decision to seek professional health care.

Table 4.1 illustrates how those people whose ideas of health and illness are compatible with those of health professionals and who live within close knit communities are most likely to use professional health services. Conversely, those people living in close-

Table 4.1 Uptake of health services as influenced by the Lay Referral System (adapted from Freidson, 1970)

Lay referral structure	Lay culture	
	Compatible with profession	Incompatible with profession
Transitory	Medium to high use of services	Medium to low use of services
Stable	Highest use of services	Lowest use of services

knit communities but whose conceptions of health and illness differ from those of health professionals are least likely to use services. In transient communities – that is, communities whose members are constantly changing – where beliefs regarding health and illness are congruent with official notions of health, there is still a high degree of utilisation; but it is noticeably lower in such communities where people's conceptions are at odds with those of health care practitioners.

An example of the lay referral system, as proposed by Freidson, was found in a study of the use of maternity services by working-class mothers in Aberdeen (Mckinlay, 1973). Those mothers who had relatives living close by and who visited friends frequently were found to be under-utilisers of health care services, whereas those mothers who lived more closely to friends rather than relatives, and who had more friends of their own age, were found to be service users. This latter group were found to make considerable use of friends and husbands and consulted less with their mothers and other relatives on matters of health. Moreover, they consulted with a narrow range of lay persons. In other words, women with immediate family ties consulted less with the health care services than women who were more reliant on friends. A person's immediate social environment, the composition of family and friendship networks, then, can play a significant role in determining the frequency with which health professionals will be consulted.

LAY HEALTH CARE WORKERS

We can all be considered 'health workers' in as much as we will, at some time or another, be responsible for the health of ourselves and for others. The idea that we may be involved in the provision of health care is easier to appreciate if we consider a broader notion of health care than has hitherto been the norm. For example, self-care such as cleaning our teeth, eating a healthy diet and taking exercise, can be conceived of as health care. Looking after family and friends is also an important aspect of health care. Indeed, such informal carers, the majority of whom are unpaid, comprise a very significant proportion of health workers in our society. As we discussed in the previous chapter health care work for chronic conditions can encompass social, psychological and technological aspects of care. Technological and therapeutic aspects of care can comprise using and administering specialised equipment or drugs. For example, learning how to use an inhaler for the treatment of asthma, using a kidney dialysis machine in renal failure, or the self-monitoring of blood sugar levels for the management of diabetes. A study of young people's use of chelation therapy (the nightly infusion of an agent, through an operating pump, to remove excess iron), which forms part of their treatment regimen for the condition *thalas-saemia major,* illustrates the extent and sophistication of routine lay health care work that may be undertaken by both parents and children (Atkin and Ahmad, 2002). However, this study also reveals how compliance with the therapy is especially problematic for teenagers who very often are keen to rebel against those in authority, such as parents and doctors. Thus we see again that health care routines, mesh with other routines that are part and parcel of everyday life.

Stacey (1988) has argued in her book, *The Sociology of Health and Healing*:

1. That all members of society are actively involved in health pro-duction and maintenance work.
2. That everyone is potentially involved in health work as a patient, and that the patient is a health worker.
3. That more people than the official recognised healers are health workers.
4. That the characteristics of 'human service' or 'people work' involved in health work result in the activity having character-istics which distinguish it from most other social activities.

In addition to traditional health care workers such as general practitioners, dentists and nurses, the community pharmacist is also in regular communication with other health workers, includ-ing people who are practising self-care, and people such as parents, friends and relatives who are caring for others. Moreover, our society depends on these workers or unpaid carers and they have been referred to as the *'hidden labour of the NHS'* (Taylor, 1979). The changing demographic structure of our society, with increasing numbers of people living beyond 65, has not been matched by a corresponding increase in the funding for the provi-sion of care to the community. This has led to a growing depend-ency on family and friends for the care of elderly relatives, who are likely to have multiple medical conditions requiring poten-tially complex medication regimes (Allen, 1985). There are cur-rently an estimated 5.7 million such informal carers in Britain, with half of these caring for people aged 75 years or older (Office for National Statistics, 1998). Carers undertake a range of medication-related activities on behalf of the care-recipient, including contact with GP surgeries and pharmacies, collecting prescriptions and medication, clinical decision-making and medi-cine administration (Francis *et al.*, 2002; Gupta *et al.*, 2002). Carers require information and support dependent upon their level of responsibility for the care-recipient's medication. However, evid-ence suggests that carers may lack the appropriate medicines-related knowledge, and experience problems accessing medical and pharmaceutical services (Goldstein and Rivers, 1996). Clearly, pharmacists have an important role in ensuring that the information and service needs of both carer and care-recipient are met appropriately, though they must also be cognisant of the care-recipient's rights to autonomy and confidentiality (Francis *et al.*, 2002).

THE SICK ROLE

In the preceding chapter we suggested that what constitutes 'normality' is socially specific. In other words what is considered normal varies between societies and between groups within society. Following on from the appreciation of this, illness has been conceived by some sociologists as a 'deviant' state, in that to be ill implies a departure from normality. The notion of illness as deviance developed in the 1950s out of critiques of the biomedical model of illness which explained illness behaviour purely as a breakdown of the normal functioning of the body.

The work of an American sociologist, Talcott Parsons (1902–79), is prominent among these critiques. Parsons (1951) defined illness not as a biological state but as a social role – namely, the 'sick role'. This role distinguishes those who are healthy from those that society, and the medical profession in particular, classifies as being ill. The purpose of this distinction, Parsons argues, is to ensure the cohesion and stability of society. In playing out our everyday conventional roles – for example, as employees or employers, as unemployed, as members of families, or as pensioners – the social order is maintained. These roles, he argues, have a positive and purposeful function in maintaining the social order. Taking on roles which are not conventional – for example, that of a criminal or 'drop out' – undermines the social order and is generally considered deviant behaviour because conventional roles are not being filled.

The 'sick role' maintains the cohesion of society since those who are incapacitated are granted the privilege of having their conventional day-to-day responsibilities and duties suspended in order to allow them to restore themselves to health and expedite their return back into the social system, with its obligations, duties and roles.

In Western society only a medical practitioner can legitimise entry into the sick role. Once admitted to this role, the patient gains two benefits:

1. Patients are temporarily excused their normal roles. Gaining a sickness certificate from the doctor is the obvious way in which this expectation is met. Merely visiting the doctor, however, confers some legitimacy on the claim to be sick. Whereas 'feeling unwell' might be treated sceptically by friends and

colleagues, a visit to the doctor may be sufficient to gain credibility.

2. Patients are not held responsible for their illness. Not being held responsible for the illness relieves the patient of a considerable burden in our society. In some other societies the patient may be held responsible in that, for example, the illness may be believed to be a punishment for some past crime, sin or transgression.

However, in return for these benefits, patients are in turn expected to fulfil two obligations:

1. Patients must want to get well and should recognise that the sick role is only a temporary state which they must want to leave behind. If they apparently do not want to get well then instead of the sick role being conferred by the doctor, they may be categorised as malingerers or hypochondriacs.
2. Patients must co-operate with technically competent help. The fact that it is only medical practitioners who can legitimately confer the sick role in our society ensures that the technically competent help tends to be confined to the official medical services. Patients who choose to defer to a lay person with claims to medical knowledge, in preference to a medical practitioner, are judged as not fulfilling one of the basic obligations of the sick role.

The patient's 'sick role', along with the professional role of the doctor in this relationship as suggested by Parsons, is summarised in Table 4.2.

Critics of Parsons' concept of the 'sick role' have taken him to task over its rigidity. Indeed, we have already illustrated that help-seeking is problematic and we cannot always assume that the presence of symptoms leads to a demand for professional help. Kassebaum and Baumann (1965) have shown that the perception of illness and the subsequent routes to help-seeking varied between different ethnic groups, whilst in a study of New York residents a great deal of variation in their expectations of the sick role was identified (Gordon, 1966). Further, although the notion of the sick role is undoubtedly very useful in explaining illness behaviour for some people, particularly those with acute conditions, individuals with chronic conditions, and those with conditions having no immediately obvious cause (for example, *myalgic encephalomyelitis* [M.E.]), might not be seen to be eligible for assignation to the sick role. This is further complicated because the division between health and sickness may be blurred, the diagnosis and prognosis may be uncertain, and it may not be clear what actions the patient can or should adopt to get well. This failure to encompass those with long-term chronic illness may

Patient: sick role Obligations and privileges	Doctor: professional role Expected to:
1. Must want to get well as quickly as possible	1. Apply a high degree of skill and knowledge to the problem of illness
2. Should seek professional medical advice and co-operate with the doctor	2. Act for the welfare of the patient and community rather for their own self-interest, desire for money, advancement, etc.
3. Allowed (and may be expected) to shed some normal activities and responsibilities (e.g. employment, household tasks)	3. Be objective and emotionally detached (i.e. should not judge patients' behaviour in terms of personal value system or become emotionally involved with them)
4. Regarded as being in need of care and unable to get better by his or her own decision and will	4. Be guided by rules of professional practice
	Rights: 1. Granted the right to examine patients physically and to enquire into intimate areas of physical and personal life
	2. Granted considerable autonomy in professional practice
	3. Occupies position of authority in relation to the patient

Table 4.2 Analysis of the roles of patients and doctors, as suggested by Parsons (reproduced with permission from Patrick and Scambler, 1986)

explain why doctors tend to be better disposed to those 'acute' specialities, such as general medicine and surgery, compared with those dealing with chronic problems.

Other critics have argued that Parsons' sick role is biased in favour of the medical profession. That is, the definition of illness which authorises entry to this role is the definition of the medical profession, not that of the patient, and as such cannot adequately account for the patient's attitudes, beliefs and experiences, all of which contribute towards illness behaviour (Mechanic and Volkart, 1960). This particular criticism has focused attention on the process which leads the patient to consult with a doctor. Freidson (1961, 1970) argues that prior to consulting with a doctor, patients who experience symptoms initially discuss them with friends, relatives or colleagues. It is this referral group, rather than the medical profession, which, Freidson argues, defines the individual's experience of symptoms as illness. Consequently, a distinction has been suggested between the 'sick role' (sickness initially being defined by friends, relatives and colleagues) and the 'patient role' (concerning the role of the patients as defined by doctors).

In spite of the sick role's shortcomings, it does, nonetheless, highlight the fact that sickness is an active social role rather than a passive biological state. Moreover, since Parsons' sick role is an ideal type, it provides a model against which we can measure actual illness behaviour and experience (Nettleton, 1995). For instance, we can see how pharmacists, through responding to symptoms, counter-prescribing medicines, providing advice and referring individuals to other health practitioners contribute to the sick role by sanctioning illness and providing the public with the means, through appropriate treatment, to leave that role.

Significantly, Parsons' concept of the sick role was established during an era characterised by a paternalistic model of health care, in which 'compliant' patients were relatively powerless in the face of medical expertise. Over the past decades it has become clear that a whole range of professional–client relationships may exist, with the patient's role ranging from that of passive to active participant in decision-making, with scope for tension and dis-agreement (see below). In contemporary British society indi-viduals are increasingly asked to take responsibility for their own health, and health professionals have subscribed to the notion of concordance in which *the work of the prescriber and patient in the consultation is a negotiation between equals . . . This alliance, may, in the end, include an agreement to differ'* (Royal Pharmaceutical Society of Great Britain, 1997).

It should also be recognised that the tendency of commentators and researchers to talk nowadays of 'patient empowerment', 'expert patients' and patients as 'health consumers' may be overly simplistic. Patients may be unable or unwilling to assume the role of 'health consumer' or to challenge a health professional's authority. Some may prefer instead to remain passive in their encounters with health professionals. Consequently, much illness is still largely treated in accordance with the Parsonian model (Lupton, 2002).

RELATIONSHIPS BETWEEN PATIENTS AND HEALTH CARE PROFESSIONALS

Pharmacists are being encouraged to communicate with patients, and patients are encouraged to seek advice from their pharmacist. So what form might the relationship between patients and phar-macists take? There have been relatively few detailed sociological studies of the interactions between pharmacists and patients. The general practitioner–patient relationship, however, has been extensively studied in medical sociology and we shall consider this literature because it is likely to have implications for other health professions.

We have already discussed Parsons' work on the 'sick role', which has defined the respective roles of patient and doctor. As conceived by Parsons, the interaction between health professionals and patients comprises what may be termed a consensual relationship. That is to say, that the relationship between the two is one of stable interaction, with both participants assuming shared expectations and values. According to Parsons, such values are internalised through the process of socialisation. Consequently, society is seen to function harmoniously: the medical profession serves the functions of treating and legitimising illness, whilst patients acknowledge the authority of the medical profession to do so – that is, the doctor–patient relationship is reciprocal in nature.

The consensus approach to professional–patient relationships was developed by Szasz and Hollender (1956). They identified three different forms that the relationship might take, although they still assumed an essentially reciprocal relationship (Table 4.3).

As can be seen from Table 4.3, Szasz and Hollender describe three types of consultation:

1. The activity/passivity relationship, where the patient passively receives treatment (for example in the operating theatre).
2. The guidance/co-operation relationship, where the doctor tells the patient what to do in the case of acute illness (for example, the treatment of an infection).
3. The mutual participation relationship, where the doctor helps the patient to help him or herself (for example, modification of diet in the treatment of obesity).

We might suppose the mutual participation model would be the most appropriate to describe the community pharmacist–client relationship because, as we have seen, patients are encouraged to seek health care advice from pharmacists so that they can practise self-care. The consensus approach to the doctor–patient relationship

Table 4.3 Szasz and Hollender's three models of patient–health professional relationship (reproduced with permission from Patrick and Scambler, 1986)

Model	Doctor's role	Patient's role
Activity/passivity	Does something to the patient	Recipient (unable to respond)
Guidance/co-operation (obeys)	Tells patient what to do	Co-operation
Mutual participation	Helps patients to help themselves	Participant in 'partnership'

always assumes the health professional to be an authority and the patient is content to be deferential. However, it has been argued that we cannot assume reciprocity, nor can we assume a shared system of values and expectations. In contrast to the consensus model, we must also consider conflict models. Freidson, for example, saw inherent in the professional–patient relationship a 'clash of perspectives'. The health professional and the patient have different values, ideas, priorities, interests, goals and knowledge. Indeed, as we have seen, lay people often have elaborate ideas on the causes of illness which, whilst they are inherently rational, may not necessarily match those of the medical profession. Consequently, Freidson (1975) has noted that *'the separate worlds of experience and reference of the lay person and of the professional worker are always in potential conflict with each other'*.

Bloor and Horobin (1975) see that conflict is implicit in the doctor–patient relationship. They point out that *'the sick person is first encouraged to participate in and then excluded from the therapeutic process'*. Parsons' assumption of reciprocity is thus suspect. Patients are encouraged to assess their own symptoms accurately and yet adopt a passive and deferential role once they enter the surgery. This places the patient in what Bloor and Horobin refer to as a 'double bind situation'.

Doctors are undoubtedly in a more powerful position during the consultation than the patient because of their social status and prestige. They are able to control the events in the surgery and so there is very rarely open conflict between the two parties. However, whilst doctors may appear to be in authority the patients may not necessarily be wholly passive. Stimson and Webb (1975), in their book *Going to the Doctor*, have illustrated how patients may in fact practise subtle forms of negotiation with the doctor during the consultation.

Concordance

The Concordance Initiative (see also Chapter 8) is a response to the changed relationship between the public and health professionals. Whereas in the past, doctors and pharmacists told individuals how to take their medicines correctly, now the public may be actively invited to participate in the decision-making process regarding medicines use. While historically services were accessed under a patronage system in which the public's role was to remain passive and undemanding in the process of receiving care, today patients are more likely to be actively involved in the process and inclined to be questioning and demanding. In this respect we might talk not of patients but rather of consumers or users of health services. This change in the nature of the relationship between the public and health professionals is exemplified by the concept of 'concordance', which is a term used to denote the degree to which patients and health care practitioners agree about the nature of illness and the need for treatment (Horne, 2001). Concordance is used as an alternative (though not with exactly the same meaning) to 'compliance' or 'adherence' which described whether patients received the correct medication at the correct dose and correct time, as delineated by a health professional. As such, these terms have been criticised as relating to a situation in which patients are expected to 'comply' with a practitioner's orders. A report by the Royal Pharmaceutical Society of Great Britain (1997), supported by the Department of Health, promoted the concept of 'concordance' to pharmacists and other health professionals, recognising that patients were more likely to take their medicines appropriately, if they and health professionals were in agreement about the nature of illness and the relative benefits and risks of any proposed treatments.

While the development of the public as consumers of health services may liberate them from their relatively powerless position in their encounters with health care providers, functioning in a more assertive manner also requires individuals to assume a greater responsibility for their own health. Therefore, increasingly, health care consumers are required to make decisions regarding their health on the basis of assessing risk (see Chapter 1). For example, deciding whether or not to immunise against diseases is a decision based on risk assessment. Similarly, deciding whether to begin taking medication or complete a course of medication after symptoms disappear also involves making a decision on the basis of assessing the risk associated with this behaviour. A central tenet of the concept of risk is that we as a population are always potentially at risk of illness.

The 'expert patient'

Whilst health professionals retain power and prestige in relation to the public they serve, it is undoubtedly true that in recent years the professional–patient relationship has undergone considerable change. Previously patients were presumed to be passive participants, and health care providers were perceived as repositories of expert knowledge and were treated with deference and respect. As we have seen, however, research has revealed that this was never an accurate description of patients and lay people, who in fact have long taken an active interest in their own health and health care. Nevertheless, nowadays specialist knowledge is more readily available to all, most notably through the media and Internet, and patients may have greater detailed understanding of their particular condition than the practitioners with whom they come into contact, and are aware of the risks to health associated with their condition. Governments are keen to capitalise on this expertise and this has recently resulted in the concept of the *'expert patient'*. The Department of Health report 'The Expert Patient – a New Approach to Chronic Disease Management for the 21st Century' (www.ohn.gov.uk/ohn/people/expert.htm) states that:

'The era of the patient as the passive recipient of care is being replaced by a new emphasis on the relationship between the NHS and the people whom it serves – one in which health professionals and patients are genuine partners seeking together the best solutions to each patient's problems.'

CONSULTING A GENERAL PRACTITIONER

A person is likely to consult a health professional when the perceived benefits to them outweigh the perceived costs. A visit to the general practitioner might include three potential benefits:

1. People frequently visit their general practitioner because they hope that he or she will be able to provide treatment which will alleviate their symptoms. The general practitioner may be able to make a diagnosis, indicate a prognosis, and offer treatment accordingly. Many cases, however, are not so clear-cut and a degree of uncertainty enters into the consultation – this is often the case where the doctor, who is working within the medical model of health and disease (Chapter 5), cannot find a pathological cause for a problem.
2. Visiting a general practitioner may legitimise one's status as a patient and permit entry into the 'sick role'. An obvious example of this is where employers require a 'sick note' that confirms the employee's 'illness', or in the case of welfare benefits which are only granted on the basis of a doctor's decision. The doctor has, as we have seen, the social and legal authority to grant this status.
3. A visit to the doctor may arise out of uncertainty or anxiety about certain physical or mental states and a patient may seek reassurances that their 'condition' is neither harmful nor abnormal. Because of the social prestige granted to doctors, some people may feel that the doctor can offer sound advice on aspects of their social lives, social relationships, and so on.

Some critics have argued that such growing dependency on doctors is a detrimental side effect of that profession's monopoly over health and illness (Zola, 1973; Illich, 1974).

CONSULTING A PHARMACIST

In seeking to acquire professional health care, a patient having a particularly acute symptom, such as a growth or severe bleeding, will almost invariably consult a hospital or community based medical practitioner. An individual with a mild symptom such as sunburn, an insect bite reaction, a hangover or slight graze or cut may be inclined to consult a pharmacist (though as we have seen in Chapter 3 many factors will be involved before a patient ultimately presents a symptom to a pharmacist or indeed any other health professional). These examples of acute and minor symptoms could be said to represent the extremes of a spectrum of symptoms. Between them there are a large number and range of symptoms which both general practitioners and pharmacists may be capable of dealing with. However, it would seem reasonable to speculate that symptoms which are perceived by the individual to be relatively trivial are more likely to be presented to the pharmacist than symptoms perceived to be severe. The pharmacist can therefore offer appropriate treatment and advice for such minor ailments. Beyond diagnosis and treatment of minor ailments, pharmacists offer the public several other services:

1. *Confirmation of health status.* The concept of 'illness behaviour' has been offered to explain the changes in behaviour associated with becoming ill (see Chapter 3). Though the doctor plays a fundamental role in assisting the transition from 'person' to 'patient' the pharmacist often facilitates the change by giving credibility to the individual's symptoms as serious enough to warrant the attention of the doctor. Instructions by pharmacists on how to administer prescribed medicines consolidates this change in status from person to patient by reinforcing the message that being ill requires compliance with the instruction of health care professionals. The doctor may tell a patient to take plenty of rest as part of the treatment regimen while the pharmacist might inform the patient on the consequences of non-compliance with the prescribed regimen. More often, however, people adopt different behaviour patterns which ease their transition from person to patient. Additionally, by confirming a person's status as 'unwell' the pharmacist can confirm that the patient has a legitimate claim to the general practitioner's time.

2. *Availability and accessibility.* The decision to consult a general practitioner involves a process of weighing up the costs and benefits to the patient. Costs such as loss of earnings, time and arranging an appointment may or may not outweigh any perceived benefits. Consultations in a pharmacy require no prior appointment, and pharmacies are available in most communities. The accessibility and ready availability of both the pharmacist and counter staff (often trained) provide unparalleled service for opportunistic health care advice and treatment. Patients do not have to register with a pharmacist, unlike with a general practitioner or dentist. Patients therefore can choose which pharmacist to consult, and may do so on the basis of

gender, ethnicity and age. This may be a particular advantage when seeking advice, for example, about sexual health, family planning, menstruation, laxatives and haemorrhoids.

3. *Information source and supplier of both conventional and unorthodox treatments.* Pharmacies are major suppliers of conventional medicines to the public. Moreover, pharmacists are a ready source of information about unorthodox medical therapies, such as homeopathy, vitamins, health foods, and herbal remedies. If this information is to be perceived as impartial, it is essential that pharmacists retain their professional integrity (Chapter 7). Pharmacists are in the business of selling health care products and treatments and so there is the potential here for them to be influenced by both commercial interests and their need to run a profitable business. However, in being seen to act in the best interests of their clients they can provide impartial and increasingly evidence-based advice, and as such counter the often 'inflated' claims made, in media advertising, for both conventional and complementary therapies.

4. *Major source for dispensing prescriptions.* The vast majority (95 per cent) of all prescriptions in Great Britain are dispensed from a pharmacy (the remainder being accounted for by dispensing doctors). Consequently, patients (or their relatives or carers) are most likely to visit a pharmacy in addition to having consulted the prescriber. This provides the opportunity for patients to seek clarification on their medication and discuss related or indeed unrelated health matters.

5. *Health promotion and diagnostic testing.* Pharmacists can engage in health promotion activities on a range of health related issues, such as nutrition, smoking cessation and drug misuse. This aspect of pharmacists' activities is discussed in detail in Chapter 8. Pharmacists may also provide a range of diagnostic services from their pharmacies, which can be seen as contributing to their profile of community-based heath promoter. Such services include blood sugar and cholesterol measurement, blood pressure monitoring and pregnancy testing.

SUMMARY

- Pharmacists are ideally located to provide information and support about a wide range of health issues, 'diagnosing' and treating minor ailments
- Where appropriate, pharmacists refer health service users to other health professionals, and offer support to people who have expertise in managing their own illness
- Seeking help from a health professional may be a complex social process. Certain events may 'trigger' people proactively to seek help.

- Lay people undertake health care work which may range from simple self care to using complex technologies and administering drug regimens
- The 'sick role' is a key concept which identifies the rights and responsibilities of both patients and health professionals. Although rather dated, it can still be instructive for understanding the nature of professional–patient interactions
- The term 'concordance' refers to they way in which health professionals are encouraged to see their patients or clients as 'experts' with whom they may openly discuss and negotiate treatments so that they may come to an agreement about the appropriate course of action
- We have seen that an individual's response to ill-health and consultation with a health professional is a social process. This is summarised in Figure 4.1.

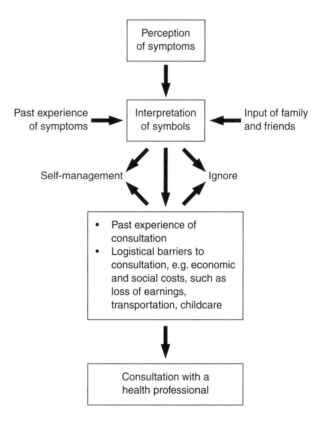

Figure 4.1
Consultation as a social process

Further reading

Albrecht, G.L., Fitzpatrick, R. and Scrimshaw, S.C. (2000) *The Handbook of Social Studies in Health and Medicine*, London, Sage.

Bissell, P., Traulsen, J.M. and Haugbølle, L.S. (2002) An introduction to functionalist sociology: Talcott Parsons' concept of the 'sick role'. *International Journal of Pharmacy Practice*, 10, 60–68.

Clark, A. (2001) *The Sociology of Health Care*, London, Prentice-Hall.

References

Allen, G. (1985) *Family Life: Domestic Roles and Social Organisation*, Oxford, Basil Blackwell.

Atkin, K. and Ahmad, W.I.U. (2002) Pumping iron: compliance with chelation therapy among young people who have thalassaemia major. In: S. Nettleton and U. Gustafsson (eds) *The Sociology of Health and Illness Reader*, Cambridge, Polity Press, pp. 223–233.

Bloor, M. and Horobin, G. (1975) Conflict and conflict resolution in doctor–patient interactions. In: C. Cox and M.E. Mead (eds) *A Sociology of Medical Practice*, London, Collier-Macmillan, pp. 271–285.

British Market Research Bureau Ltd (1997) *Everyday Healthcare Study of Self-medication in Great Britain*, London, The Proprietary Association of Great Britain.

Cartwright, A. and Anderson, R. (1981) *General Practice Revisited: A Second Study of Patients and their Doctors*, London, Tavistock Publications.

Francis, S.-A., Smith, F., Gray, N. and Graffy, J. (2002) The roles of informal carers in the management of medication for older care recipients. *International Journal of Pharmacy Practice*, 10, 1–9.

Freidson, E. (1961) *Patients' Views of Medical Practice*, New York, Russell Sage Foundation.

Freidson, E. (1970) *Profession of Medicine, a Study of the Sociology of Applied Knowledge*, New York, Harper Row.

Freidson, E. (1975) Dilemmas in the doctor–patient relationship. In: C. Cox and M.E. Mead (eds) *A Sociology of Medical Practice*, London, Collier-Macmillan, pp. 285–298.

Goldstein, R. and Rivers, P. (1996) The medication role of informal carers. *Health and Social Care in the Community*, 4, 150–158.

Gordon, G. (1966) *Role Theory and Illness: A Sociological Perspective*, New Haven, Conn., College and University Press.

Gupta, D., Smith, F. and Francis, S.-A. (2002) Investigating medicines-related roles and problems experienced by informal careers of older patients. *Hospital Pharmacist*, 9, 55–58.

Horne, R. (2001) Compliance, adherence and concordance. In: K.M.G. Taylor and G. Harding (eds) *Pharmacy Practice*, London, Taylor and Francis, pp. 165–184.

Illich, I. (1974) *Medical Nemesis*, London, Calder Boyars.

Kassebaum, G.G. and Baumann, B.O. (1965) Dimensions of the sick role in chronic illness. *Journal of Health and Human Behaviour*, 6, 16–27.

Lupton, D. (2002) Consumerism, reflexivity and the medical encounter. In: S. Nettleton and U. Gustafsson (eds) *The Sociology of Health and Illness Reader*, Cambridge, Polity Press, pp. 360–368.

Mckinlay, J.B. (1973) Social networks, lay consultations and help-seeking behaviour. *Social Forces*, 51, 255–292.

Mechanic, D. and Volkart, E. (1960) Illness behaviour and medical diagnosis. *Journal of Health and Human Behaviour*, 1, 86–94.

Nettleton, S. (1995) *The Sociology of Health and Illness*, Cambridge, Polity Press.

Office for National Statistics (1998) *Informal Carers*, London, Office for National Statistics.

Parsons, T. (1951) *The Social System*, London, Free Press.

Patrick, D. and Scambler, G. (eds) (1986) *Sociology as Applied to Medicine*, London, Bailliere Tindall.

Royal Pharmaceutical Society of Great Britain (1997) *From Compliance to Concordance: Achieving Shared Goals in Medicine Taking*, London, Royal Pharmaceutical Society of Great Britain.

Stacey, M. (1988) *The Sociology of Health and Healing*, London, Unwin Hyman.

Stimson, G.V. and Webb, B. (1975) *Going to See the Doctor*, London, Routledge and Kegan Paul.

Szasz, T.S. and Hollender, M.H. (1956) A contribution to the philosophy of medicine: the basic models of the doctor–patient relationship. *Archives of International Medicine*, 97, 585–592.

Taylor, J. (1979) Hidden labour in the national health service. In: P. Atkinson, R. Dingwall and A. Murcott (eds) *Prospects for National Health*, London, Croom Helm.

Zola, I.K. (1973) Pathways to the doctor: from person to patient. *Social Science and Medicine*, 7, 677–689.

5 Social Factors and Health

INTRODUCTION

In this chapter we introduce the idea that there is relationship between social factors and health. Within the social sciences there is a long tradition of research which has sought to identify those factors which influence health status. Sociologists have worked together with epidemiologists to study the social distribution of health and illness, and the social determinants of diseases. (The findings of this research are discussed more fully in Chapter 6.) We will first discuss the possibilities and problems associated with measuring health and illness. We will then illustrate how historical epidemiological studies have revealed how the influence of bio-medicine for the improvement of health has been overplayed. These studies have contributed to the consolidation of two contrasting perspectives or models of health and illness: namely, the medical/bio-medical model and the social models.

MEASURING HEALTH

Measures of health, illness and disease are notoriously complex. Traditionally the key measures of health status and health 'outcome' have been measures of mortality (death) and morbidity (disease). Today, however, epidemiologists, health service researchers and social sciences can draw on a vast array of tools and techniques for measuring what are sometimes referred to as the 'five D's': death, disease, disability, discomfort and dissatisfaction (Fitzpatrick, 1997). We can see from this list that what we need to measure is not necessarily straightforward and will depend on how we define these terms. For example, how would we measure discomfort? Should it be based upon the patient's perspective, a clinician's assessment or a set of physical criteria? In practice, measurement instruments have been developed to capture all of these. For example, simple and subjective self-report measures are often based upon questionnaires designed to capture patients' views. Measures of functioning can assess physical capacity, and quality of life instruments assess the impact of disease, illness or impairment on people's lives. We do not intend to provide a detailed discussion of these measures here as they can be found elsewhere (Bowling, 1995, 1997). The burgeoning of health and illness measures is part and parcel of the shift from a bio-medical model of health and illness, which focuses upon the pathological nature of disease, to the social model of health and illness, which takes a wider view and attempts to understand the social determinants and social consequences of health and illness. We return to these models of health below, but first let us consider the most common measures of health status – namely, mortality and morbidity. We will see that data using these measures have yielded valuable evidence of the inequitable distribution of health chances in the community. However, it should be appreciated that even these measures are inherently problematic.

It is important that we clarify what is meant by these epidemiological indicators.

Mortality rates

Mortality or death rates are usually presented as the number of deaths per 1,000 living members of a population per year. The crude death rate will be affected by the demographic composition of the population. Therefore age-specific death rates can be calculated thus:

$$\frac{\text{number of deaths of a given age} \times 1,000}{\text{number in population at that age}}$$

These may also be calculated separately for men and women and for different occupational categories, and are then termed 'standardised' death or mortality rates. The standardised mortality rate is a method of comparing death rates between different sections of the population holding other variables constant, i.e. comparing one area with another, whilst holding age, sex and occupation constant.

Mortality rates which are regarded to be particularly important indicators of social welfare, circumstances and health status are the neonatal, perinatal and infant mortality rates.

Neonatal mortality rate

$$\frac{\text{Deaths at 0–27 days after live birth} \times 1,000}{\text{Live births}}$$

Perinatal mortality rate

$$\frac{\text{Stillbirths} + \text{deaths at 0–6 days after live birth} \times 1,000}{\text{Live births} + \text{stillbirths}}$$

Infant mortality rate

$$\frac{\text{Deaths under the age of one year after live birth} \times 1,000}{\text{Live births}}$$

Morbidity incidence, prevalence and rates

Morbidity refers to sickness or disease. The incidence of a disease is the number of times it occurs, i.e. the number of cases contracted or resulting in death, in a given social group within a given period of time, e.g. how many new cases are reported in a year. The prevalence of a disease is the total number of cases, i.e. the number of people suffering from the disease in a given time.

The distribution of disease in different populations may be adjusted to take into account the size of the population. This process results in ratios where the number of cases of the disease (the prevalence or incidence) is divided by the number of people in the population. Because these ratios often result in very small numbers the ratio is multiplied by 1,000. This has the effect of producing a ratio which indicates how many cases of disease exist per 1,000. The morbidity rate is thus:

$$\frac{\text{Number of people with disease in the population} \times 1,000}{\text{Number of people in the population}}$$

Rates may be further calculated for specific sub-groups, for example to produce age-specific, sex-specific or occupation-specific morbidity rates.

MacIntyre (1988) has highlighted some problems associated with using mortality and morbidity rates as indicators of health. She points out that mortality rates are increasingly unreliable because:

1. Reductions of mortality rates to low levels in industrialised countries make comparisons unreliable because of the small numbers involved.
2. With the overall increase in life expectancy and a considerably smaller proportion of deaths occurring before the age of 65 years than in the past, data on those who are economically active are based on a smaller proportion of the total population than in the past.
3. Mortality rates clearly cannot measure improvement, stability or deterioration in health.
4. Mortality rates are based on a binary division of dead or alive and therefore they are not sensitive to degrees of healthiness of those still alive.
5. With changes in the nature of disease, i.e. with an increase in chronic and degenerative diseases and the overall decrease in infectious diseases, mortality rates are less useful because, although they are falling, morbidity may at the same time be increasing.
6. Morbidity rates and mortality rates have sometimes been found

to be at odds for certain social groups; for example, women live longer than men yet have higher rates of morbidity.

MacIntyre (1988) has also set out the shortcomings of morbidity measures:

1. Morbidity measures which are based on the uptake of health services – that is, how many people use a given service (for example, visit their general practitioner) – are often used as indicators of morbidity. However, such measures may tell us more about the nature and availability of service provision than about morbidity *per se*.
2. Self-reported data of health are based on the individual's concepts and perceptions of symptoms and illness. Clearly interpretations of these may vary between groups which the researcher might be seeking to compare.
3. There are known variations in diagnostic conventions between countries and these also change over time, potentially making comparisons between time and place unreliable.

These difficulties encountered in measuring health do not imply that the existing data have no value. Rather, in drawing attention to these difficulties, we are seeking to emphasise the nature of the subject matter we hope to understand. We must be constantly vigilant in our methods of collecting and interpreting data because the social world, by its very nature, cannot be explained or understood by definite concepts or static measures. We can see that health, illness and disease are not neat and tidy variables, which are easily measured. Our appreciation of this has contributed to the recognition that they are not objective concepts that can be understood in isolation from the social context.

PERSPECTIVES ON HEALTH AND DISEASE

During the last few decades there has been a transformation in the way certain elements of medicine and medical practice are comprehended. The academic disciplines of medical sociology and epidemiology, along with social movements such as consumer groups and women's movements and the growth of interest in complementary medicine, have begun to challenge orthodox medical ideas; in particular, they have challenged bio-medical explanations of the causes of disease.

The medical model of health and disease

In the nineteenth and early twentieth centuries, disease was believed to be the direct consequence of specific causal agents such as bacteria or viruses. The 'germ theory' of disease came to be the main form of explanation in scientific medicine, and is sometimes referred to as the *'doctrine of specific aetiology'* (Dubos, 1959). It constituted the dominant intellectual framework or 'paradigm' within which medicine worked, and this framework has been loosely termed the 'medical' or 'bio-medical' model. This model represents a set of basic assumptions held by medical scientists about the nature and causes of health and disease. These assumptions include:

1. That all disease can be traced to a specific aetiology such as a virus, parasite or bacterium.
2. That the patient's body can be treated like a machine in that during treatment it is passive, and can be made better through medical 'engineering'.
3. That the elimination of disease and the return to health depend on medical technology and/or chemical intervention.

The socio-environmental model of health and disease

The 'socio-environmental' model of health and disease involves a change of emphasis from that of the medical model. Whilst the medical model emphasises the impact of medicine in the elimination of disease, the socio-environmental model emphasises the maintenance and production of good health. It also draws attention to the social causes of ill-health. All societies are stratified along cultural, religious or economic lines, and certain diseases are more prevalent among some members of a community than others. Morbidity and mortality rates are markedly influenced by predetermined factors that are social rather than genetic in character. These are represented in Figure 5.1, which illustrates that in addition to biological factors are multiple layers of factors which influence our health status.

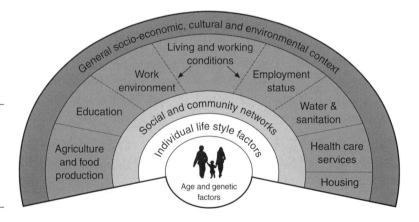

Figure 5.1 Factors impacting on health (reproduced with permission from Dahlgren and Whitehead, 1991)

Chapter Five

We can see that the 'socio-environmental model' associates disease with nutrition, hygiene, environmental and behavioural factors. An important consequence of this development has been that health cannot and should not be separated from the social environment in which a person lives. Just as the decline of infectious disease during the nineteenth century was the result of improved nutrition, hygiene and birth control, the common 'killers' of the twentieth and early twenty-first centuries – heart disease/circulatory disorders, cancer (for adults), and accidents (for children) – are all associated with factors such as occupation, stress, diet, smoking, pollution and environment. A corollary to this is that people are no longer seen as passive victims of disease but can themselves participate in the production of good health. Disease prevention is also seen to be preferable to intervention (see Chapter 8). Whilst in the medical model, health was defined by an absence of disease, a rather negative and a purely functional concept in that it implies being physically and mentally able, the socio-environmental model has yielded broader definitions of health which testify to the importance of social as well as the biophysiological perception of health (Box 5.1).

Box 5.1 Definitions of Health

WHO 1948: Health is a complete state of physical, mental and social well-being and not merely the absence of disease and infirmity.
WHO 1984: Health is the extent to which an individual or group is able, on the one hand, to realise aspirations and satisfy needs; and on the other hand, to change or cope with the environment. Health is therefore seen as a resource for everyday life, not the object of living; it is a positive concept emphasising social and personal resources, as well as physical capacities.

THE McKEOWN THESIS

In broadening the scope beyond purely biological explanations of disease to include social, environmental and psychological factors, some of the earlier claims of medicine have become subject to scrutiny. In the early 1970s an influential body of work emerged which, although originating from within the medical profession, was critical of the assumption that medical intervention alone could ameliorate disease. One such critic, McKeown (1979), by way of a complex historical demographic study illustrated that the rapid decline in the population's death rate which occurred in the eighteenth, nineteenth and twentieth centuries was due to a reduction in communicable diseases. However, this decline, he argued, had little to do with medical interventions such as immunisation programmes, but was due initially to increases in food supplies, and subsequently to better hygiene and sanitation, and to an increased acceptance of methods of birth control. Considering

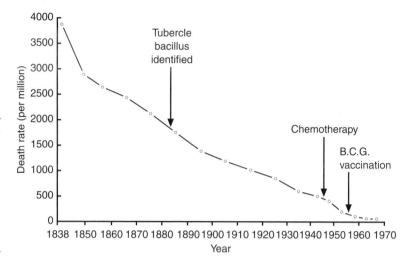

Figure 5.2 Respiratory tuberculosis: annual death rates for England and Wales 1838–1970 (reproduced with permission from McKeown, 1979)

tuberculosis as a specific example, McKeown demonstrated that a large part of the decline in the death rate from tuberculosis in England and Wales occurred before the introduction of streptomycin in 1947.

As we can see from Figure 5.2, although chemotherapeutic agents such as streptomycin markedly reduced the number of deaths between 1948 and 1970, when considered over the period from 1848 the reduction in deaths resulting from chemotherapy was less than 4 per cent. As McKeown (1979) argues,

'If we group together the advances in nutrition and hygiene as environmental measures, the influences responsible for the decline of mortality and associated improvement in health were environment, behavioural and therapeutic. They became effective from the eighteenth, nineteenth and twentieth centuries respectively and their order in time was also that of their effectiveness.'

McKeown acknowledges that medical interventions can and have been important in improving health and controlling disease. The elimination of smallpox was perhaps one of the most dramatically successful medical interventions. But his argument is that medicine's effectiveness tends to be overplayed and the contribution of medical interventions in the control of diseases is partial. Improved nutrition, change in reproduction, and improved sanitation and housing are just as important when it comes to the control and prevention of disease and illness.

The challenge to the effectiveness, appropriateness and superiority of Western medicine has been made not only by certain epidemiologists, such as McKeown, but also by other groups. Feminist sociologists, for example, have effectively demonstrated how the medical profession has only a partial understanding of health and illness and that medicine's faith in technology has, at times, blinded the profession when it comes to the type of care it offers. For instance, consider childbirth; this essentially natural process has come to be associated with a never-ending array of clinical tests, checks, screening procedures, and so on. Some more radical commentators of medicine and medical practice such as Illich (1975) have argued that medical intervention can, through its procedures, be iatrogenic (i.e. result in more harm than good).

IATROGENESIS AND MEDICINE

Illich (1975) sees the impact of medicine as being harmful on three levels; he refers to these as 'clinical', 'social' and 'cultural' iatrogenesis. Clinical iatrogenesis refers to all those conditions for which *'remedies, physicians, or hospitals are the pathogens'*; he supports his argument with data which show how drugs administered to patients have deleterious side effects on a scale that must be unacceptable, and how surgical intervention often has unintended and negative results. On the second level, medicine reinforces 'social over-medicalisation' in that more and more aspects of our lives come under the remit of medicine and in consequence many social problems are neutralised and become removed from the political arena. For example, the behaviour of delinquent children may be explained away in terms of medically defined and treated syndromes. Furthermore, Illich suggests that the presence of a medical profession which has over the past two centuries established a monopoly over medical knowledge and practice has generated a 'culture of dependence'. The lay public, Illich argues, has become reliant on medicine to the point that they no longer feel capable of caring for themselves. This dependence on so-called 'experts' constitutes cultural iatrogenesis.

Illich was not blind to the value of some clinical interventions and treatment, however. He gives the example of antibiotics as one area of medicine that was particularly successful. Today, ironically, we see that increasing use, and indeed over use of antibiotics, has led to antibiotic resistance (Humphrey, 2000) with the emergence in hospitals of so-called 'superbugs' such as *methicillin-resistant staphylococcus aureus* (MRSA).

THE COMMODIFICATION OF MEDICINE AND HEALTH

On the formation of the NHS, health care was to be free at the point of use. Health care was therefore conceptualised as a public service issue in which everyone had open and unregulated access. It soon became apparent that the demand for health services far exceeded the NHS's ability to meet and afford this demand. In recent decades, the State's response to this overwhelming demand has been to inject 'market forces' into the public health care system. This has resulted in initiatives such as the 'internal market', GP fund holding, health care trusts, etc. Commensurately, health policies have been introduced to provide a greater voice for the users of health services as exemplified by the Patient's Charter, and the overhaul of the procedures for patients to complain about the health services they receive. Increasingly then, health care services, and indeed health itself, have come to be perceived as 'commodities' within a 'marketplace' where health professionals are redefined as service providers and patients as health care consumers.

However, the commodification of health within the UK is tempered by the fact that the NHS remains a state-funded provision. Moreover, for the reasons outlined in Box 5.2, health and health care provision cannot simply be regarded as mere market commodities. Thus, in seeking the services of health professionals, the public manage a dual role: as patients dependent on professional expertise, and as consumers of this expertise with the associated rights and responsibilities.

Box 5.2 Reasons why health and health care are not simple market commodities

- Health care delivery is driven by needs, not wants
- Access to care should not be based on the ability to pay
- A privatised health care system would disadvantage patients at high risk of disease, e.g. those genetically predisposed to illness
- There is an asymmetry of expertise and power between service providers and consumers

Medicines as commodities

Historically, the public has accepted that medicines possess an inherent power to heal. Medicines were viewed as a special category of objects, having a symbolic, 'health-giving' value, reinforced by the fact that they were accessed only from a doctor's surgery or a pharmacy. This is perhaps best exemplified by the pharmacist 'making something up' within the pharmacy to treat a patient's specific symptoms. Health professionals have long claimed that the power of medicines to heal sets them apart from other objects, and that consequently they should be subject to regulatory control to prevent their inappropriate use and misuse. By controlling the public's access to pharmaceuticals the medical and pharmacy professions have acquired considerable power and prestige (see Chapter 7).

However, the public's relationship to medicines has changed and is now much more matter of fact. The range of potent medicines/pharmaceuticals available to the public over the counter rather than via a prescription has increased substantially in recent years as medicines are deregulated. Medicines previously only available on prescription can now be purchased from pharmacies, whilst those once only purchasable from pharmacies may now be found in newsagents, petrol filling stations, campsite shops, etc. Deregulation of pharmaceuticals, combined with extensive advertising and widespread availability, alters both the public's and the professionals' relations with them. General practitioners will thus advise patients who are not exempt from paying prescription charges to purchase medicines rather than access them via a prescription – demystifying, and potentially devaluing the medicines in the process. Pharmacists sell an ever-increasing range of pharmaceuticals, not as 'medicines' possessing some kind of symbolic value but rather as commodities, undifferentiated from other products. This is seen most readily in multiple and supermarket pharmacies, which with their corporate identity and ethos, advertising campaigns, self-selection merchandising, 'three for the price of two' offers and routinised sales techniques encourage pharmaceuticals to be regarded as standardised commodities, accessed in the same way as others (Harding and Taylor, 2001).

This commodification process raises specific issues, which have yet to be addressed head on, such as whether it engenders complacency with regard to overdose and adverse effects, and the removal of the public from the surveying gaze of doctors and pharmacists. However, it should be noted that whilst available as commodities, medicines can retain a high, non-pecuniary value. For example, analgesic tablets may be bought relatively cheaply as an over the counter (OTC) medicine, but as a remedy for an individual's acute symptoms they have a high value. Moreover, when that particular analgesic is specifically selected from a range of alternatives, and is endorsed by the pharmacist as being suitable for an individual's therapeutic needs, a product is 'symbolically transformed' from a mere commodity into a medicine (Harding and Taylor, 1997). This transformation is accomplished on the basis of the pharmacists' knowledge. It is not necessarily dependent upon the product's efficacy or cost, but is buttressed by professional ethics which ensure that the public's well-being takes priority over sale for profit.

THE LIMITS OF TECHNOLOGY

Pharmaceutical technology has grown apace with bio-medical technology and there is an increasing reliance today on such technology. A wide range of pharmaceutical preparations exists to treat the majority of common ailments, many of which can be bought over the counter. While this development – 'a pill for every ill' – may appear to represent a triumph of technology, increasing our reliance on technology to improve our lives, it is important to consider the limitations of technology, which encourages dependency on bio-medical science as the single authority on issues of health and healing. Indeed, in recent years considerable interest has developed in what was previously termed 'alternative medicine'. Today, 'complementary therapies' including aroma-therapy, acupuncture, homeopathy and the like, which are founded on principles other than those of bio-medical science, are increasing in popularity, possibly reflecting not simply a growing disenchantment with bio-medicine but also perhaps a recognition that bio-medicine is not invariably able to provide solutions to the problems associated with chronic illness. Thus, people seeking expert help for their health problems today increasingly turn to a range of health care providers which include complementary as well as mainstream practitioners (Cant and Sharma, 2000).

EFFECTIVENESS AND EFFICIENCY OF TREATMENT

Today, the value and effectiveness of medical technologies and therapies are not taken for granted. They are subjected to scrutiny and review – partly as a consequence of the research and critiques we have discussed above, but also because of the work of the epidemiologist and doctor Archie Cochrane. Through his work as a medical practitioner Cochrane became aware that many clinical interventions had never actually been tested or evaluated and that doctors often based their practice on their experiences rather than on any systematic evaluation of treatments. He published his views in the now influential book entitled *Effectiveness and Efficiency* (Cochrane, 1972). He subsequently developed research methods that are used to systematically collate and review research evidence on the effectiveness of interventions. The legacy of his work can be found in the Cochrane Collaboration, a network of centres throughout the world which evaluate and review evidence on health interventions. In particular, he advocated the use of randomised control trials (RCTs) as the best method for evaluating interventions.

Today this approach is summarised by the term 'evidence-based medicine'. This involves the integration of research-based information into clinical practice, and has been described thus:

'Evidence based medicine is the conscientious, explicit, and judicious use of current best evidence in making decisions about the care of individual patients. The practice of evidence based medicine means integrating individual clinical expertise with the best available external clinical evidence from systematic research ... By best available external clinical evidence we mean clinically relevant research, often from the basic sciences of

medicine, but especially from patient centred research into the accuracy and precision of diagnostic tests (including clinical examination), the power of prognostic markers, and the efficacy and safety of therapeutic, rehabilitative, and preventive regimens. External clinical evidence both invalidates previously accepted diagnostic tests and treatments and replaces them with new ones that are more powerful and accurate, more efficacious, and safer' (Sackett *et al.*, 1996).

Like physicians, pharmacists are also increasingly required to draw on evidence-based medicine as a basis for their recommendations to patients or fellow health professionals. For instance, a recent review of oral antihistamine therapy (Consumers' Association, 2002) and a randomised controlled trial of the effectiveness of pharmaceutical care in reactive airways disease (Weinberger *et al.*, 2002) are among an increasing body of published 'evidence' which has direct application to pharmacy practice.

Whilst most people would accept that the evaluation of health interventions is generally a 'good thing' the routine application of evidence-based medicine is also a source of controversy. For example, it relies on the results of collective data which a clinician might feel to be inappropriate for the individual patient with whom they are faced. Furthermore, the over-reliance on a narrow range of evidence is also criticised, in particular the over use of quantitative outcomes which may fail to grasp patients' experiences and the qualitative dimensions of patient satisfaction (Stradling and Davies, 1997). This said, qualitative methods are increasingly being incorporated into the evaluation of health and medical interventions (Green and Britten, 1998). (See also Chapter 9.)

SUMMARY

- Disease is the product of both biological and social factors
- There are two models of health and disease: namely, the medical and socio-environmental models
- Morbidity and mortality rates may be used as indicators of health status
- Medical practice can harm as well as be beneficial
- Health care and medicines are increasingly being treated as commodities, with health professionals conceptualised as service providers and patients as consumers
- The limitations of bio-medical science and medical technology have led to an increasing popularity of complementary therapies
- Health care is increasingly becoming 'evidence-based'.

FURTHER READING

Bowling, A. (1995) *Measuring Disease: A Review of Disease-Specific Quality of Life Measurement Scales*, Buckingham, Open University Press.

Bowling, A. (1997) *Measuring Health: A Review of Quality of Life Measurement Scales*, Buckingham, Open University Press.

Clarke, A. (2001) *The Sociology of Health Care*, London, Prentice-Hall.

Davey, B., Gray, A. and Seale, C. (eds) (2001) *Health and Disease: A Reader* (3rd edn), Buckingham, Open University Press.

Illich, I. (1974) *Medical Nemesis*, London, Calder Boyars.

McKeown, T. (1979) *The Role of Medicine: Dream, Mirage or Nemesis*, Oxford, Blackwell.

Sackett, D.L., Strauss, S.E., Richardson, W.S., Rosenberg, W. and Hayes, R.B. (2000) *Evidence-Based Medicine: How to Practice and Teach EBM* (2nd edn), Edinburgh, Churchill Livingstone.

REFERENCES

Bowling, A. (1995) *Measuring Disease: A Review of Disease-Specific Quality of Life Measurement Scales*, Buckingham, Open University Press.

Bowling, A. (1997) *Measuring Health: A Review of Quality of Life Measurement Scales*, Buckingham, Open University Press.

Cant, S. and Sharma, U. (2000) Alternative health practices and systems. In: G.L. Albrecht, R. Fitzpatrick and S.C. Scrimshaw (eds) *The Handbook of Social Studies in Health and Medicine*, London, Sage.

Cochrane, A. (1972) *Effectiveness and Efficiency: Random Reflections on Health Services*, London, Nuffield Provincial Hospitals Trust.

Consumers' Association (2002) *Drugs and Therapeutics Bulletin*, 40, 59–62.

Dahlgren, G. and Whitehead, M. (1991) *Policies and Strategies to Promote Social Equity in Health*, Stockholm, Institute for Futures Studies.

Dubos, R. (1959) *Mirage of Health*, New York, Harper Row.

Fitzpatrick, R. (1997) Measuring health outcomes. In: G. Scambler (ed.) *Sociology as Applied to Medicine*, London, W.B. Saunders.

Green, J. and Britten, N. (1998) *British Medical Journal*, 316, 1230–1232.

Harding, G. and Taylor, K.M.G. (1997) Responding to change: the case of community pharmacy in Britain. *Sociology of Health and Illness*, 19, 521–534.

Harding, G. and Taylor, K.M.G. (2001) McPharmacy medicines. *Pharmaceutical Journal*, 266, 56.

Humphrey, C. (2000) Antibiotic resistance: an exemplary case of medical nemesis. *Critical Public Health*, 10, 353–358.

Illich, I. (1975) *Limits to Medicine*, London, Marion Boyars.

MacIntyre, S. (1988) A review of the social patterning and significance of measures of height, weight, blood pressure, and respiratory function. *Social Science and Medicine*, 27, 327–337.

McKeown, T. (1979) *The Role of Medicine: Dream, Mirage or Nemesis*, Oxford, Blackwell.

Sackett, D.L., Rosenberg, W.M.C., Gray, J.A.M., Haynes, R.B. and Richardson, W.S. (1996) Evidence based medicine: What it is and what it isn't. It's about integrating individual clinical expertise and the best external evidence. *British Medical Journal*, 312, 71–72.

Stradling, J.R. and Davies, R. (1997) The unacceptable face of evidence based medicine. *Journal of Clinical Evaluation*, 3, 99–103.

Weinberger, M. *et al.* (2002) Effectiveness of pharmacist care for patients with reactive airways disease: a randomized controlled trial. *Journal of the American Medical Association*, 288, 1594–1602.

World Health Organisation (1948) *Official Records of the World Health Organisation, No. 2*, Geneva, World Health Organisation.

World Health Organisation (1984) *Health Promotion: A Discussion Document on the Concept and Principles*, Copenhagen, Regional Office for Europe.

6   Social Inequalities and Health

INTRODUCTION

This chapter will illustrate that health and disease are not simply biologically determined phenomena. Rather, the chances of becoming ill are frequently related to a person's social circumstances. That is to say, illness and disease are not solely associated with physiological changes but are also influenced by where we live, and how we live, work, and eat, and also by our relationships with other people. We shall examine the evidence that shows that disease has a social, as well as a biological basis – in fact, that disease is socially patterned. By this we mean that some groups of people in society are more likely to suffer from certain ailments than others. Generally the people most susceptible to ill-health are those who have the fewest material resources and who are least able to participate fully in everyday life – for example, in their access to housing, transport and employment opportunities.

Western society is manifestly unequal. People are placed hierarchically along dimensions of inequality such as age, income, occupation, gender and ethnicity, and some may subsequently suffer because of their position in society. The level at which members of a given society find themselves can influence their life chances, or their opportunities to achieve rewards, be they satisfactory careers, housing, income or health. We shall explore these dimensions of inequality in relation to health.

GENDER AND HEALTH

One important dimension of inequality is the result of social relations between men and women; that is, gender relations. Gender refers to the socially constructed differentiation between men and women, while sex refers to the biological distinction between males and females. As we shall see later in this chapter, people in higher occupational categories have social and economic advantages. Similarly, men have social and economic advantages over women. There is inequality between men and women in the family; for instance, women do more housework than men, and this is the case even when women are in full-time employment (Crompton, 1997). Similarly, domestic resources such as the family car and money are not equally shared between men and women in the same household (Miller and Glendinning, 1992). Moreover, women frequently earn less than men, and are more likely to work part-time (Evans 1998). Gender then, as a form of stratification, is of particular relevance to health and health care (Arber and Thomas, 2001).

The associations between health and gender are extremely complex. For instance, it is often claimed that there are higher rates of morbidity among women than men but that women live

Age (years)	LSLI		RA within previous 14 days	
	Males (%)	Females (%)	Males (%)	Females (%)
0–4	4	4	11	7
5–15	9	8	10	11
16–44	11	11	10	12
45–64	27	27	17	19
65–74	38	35	20	21
75+	44	48	23	27

Table 6.1 Prevalence of reported long-standing limiting illness (LSLI) and reported restricted activity (RA) within the previous fourteen days, by age and gender (reproduced with permission from Office of National Statistics, 2000)

longer. However, this idea that 'women are sicker, but men die quicker' has been challenged recently by research which has revealed that the differences in ill-health between men and women is not as great as has often been supposed (Lahelma *et al.*, 2001). As we can see from Table 6.1 the differences between men and women who report having a long-standing limiting illness, and restricted activity due to illness in the previous fourteen days, are of minor significance.

But when the social context of men and women's lives are taken into account differences do appear. For example, Lahelma and her colleagues (2001) found that women's participation in paid employment can affect their health status – women who are unemployed are likely to have worse health. Women's health is also associated with social class and ethnicity. As can be seen in Table 6.2 women in social classes IV and V have higher rates of morbidity, compared with women in other social classes. Table 6.3 reveals that such associations also interact with ethnicity. The relationships between social class, ethnicity and health are discussed more fully, as a separate issue, later in this chapter.

During the twentieth century the life expectancy of both men and women steadily increased (Table 6.4). Consistently though, women could expect to outlive men, such that currently, on average, women live six years longer. The discrepancy between the mortality and morbidity rates for men and women has been explored by sociologists. The difference may be a function of the research methods employed. For example, in studies where people report their own incidence of illness, men may be more likely to feel that illness is a sign of weakness and hence under-report the incidence of illness. Furthermore, women are found to be more predisposed to take responsibility for their health than men, explaining their (women's) higher rates of morbidity when calculated from working days lost or visits to the general practitioner.

The 'orthodoxy' that women had higher morbidity rates than men may partly have been the result of research based on health service use. Women do tend to make more use of health services – in part this may be explained by increased use for reproductive health matters such as contraception, antenatal care, and so on.

Self-reported health status	Less than good general health			Limiting long-standing illness			Large amount of stress		
	Observed (%)*	Expected (%)	Obs/exp (%)	Observed (%)*	Expected (%)	Obs/exp (%)	Observed (%)*	Expected (%)	Obs/exp (%)
Social class									
Men									
I & II	17	23	75**	17	20	84**	28	25	112**
III (Non-manual)	19	20	94	17	17	95	26	24	107
III (Manual)	26	23	113**	22	21	106	20	24	83**
IV & V	29	22	131**	25	20	126**	23	23	100
Total	22	22	100	20	20	100	24	24	100
Women									
I & II	17	24	71**	19	22	86**	35	31	116**
III (Non-manual)	24	25	96	22	23	93	27	29	92
III (Manual)	31	27	115	31	26	120	25	28	88
IV & V	33	27	123**	29	26	112**	28	29	98
Total	26	26	100	24	24	100	29	29	100

* The percentages refer to the proportions of the sub-groups reporting each health status, so do not add up to 100

** Age-standardised ratio is significantly different from 100, at the 95% level.

Table 6.2 Self-reported health status by social class based on own current or last job for men and women aged 16 and over (reproduced with permission from Rainford *et al.*, 1998)

	Self assessed health fair/poor		Activities limited by health	
	Men (%)	Women (%)	Men (%)	Women (%)
Whites	26	32	12	22
All ethnic minorities	29	35	12	19
Caribbean	33	39	8	22
All South Asians	29	33	14	18
Indian	26	32	14	15
African-Asian	26	27	10	15
Pakistani	34	38	16	24
Bangladeshi	35	41	22	21
Chinese	20	28	12	9

Table 6.3 Selected aspects of health of whites and members of ethnic minority groups (reproduced with permission of the Policy Studies Institute from Nazroo, 1997)

Table 6.4 Great Britain: life expectancy and healthy life expectancy at birth by sex (reproduced with permission from Office of National Statistics, 2001)*

Women also tend to take more care of their own health and the health of their other family members such as children, parents and their partners. The contention that women are more ill then men, but live longer, may also have been the case historically. When women's participation in the labour force was more constrained, their access to education limited and their contribution to the domestic sphere more intense, then all these factors would have compounded their health status. With social change the patterning of health and illness also changes.

In a comprehensive review of gender differences in health, Arber and Thomas (2001) identified seven kinds of explanations which have been suggested in the literature (Box 6.1). They found little evidence to support the biological and psycho-social explanations. The evidence on risk behaviours may account for the longer life expectancy of women, since they do tend to take more care of their health by eating 'healthier diets' and participating in prevention programmes. However, this would not account for their high levels of morbidity. The combined influence of the remaining four factors was found to be the most salient in accounting for women's high rates of morbidity, although their effect varies across the life-course (Macintyre *et al.*, 1996). World-wide, women are more likely to be poorer than men, have less formal education, and in both domestic and public settings have

	Years								
	1841	1901	1931	1961	1981	1986	1991	1997	1998
Males									
Life expectancy	41.0	45.7	58.1	67.8	70.9	72.0	73.2	74.6	74.9
Healthy life expectancy	–	–	–	–	64.4	65.4	66.2	66.9	–
Females									
Life expectancy	43.0	49.6	62.1	73.7	76.8	77.7	78.8	79.6	79.8
Healthy life expectancy	–	–	–	–	66.7	67.6	68.6	68.7	–

*Data for 1841 and 1901 are for England and Wales only.

Box 6.1   Explanations
of gender differences
in health (Arber and
Thomas, 2001)

1. Biological reasons
2. Psycho-social differences
3. Risk behaviours
4. Occupational and work-related factors
5. Social roles and responsibilities
6. Power and resources within the home
7. Social–structural differences within society

less power and control over their environments. Gender inequalities are compounded further by other forms of structural inequalities, such as ethnicity – to which we now turn.

ETHNICITY AND HEALTH

Another dimension of inequality in Western societies is that between the white population and ethnic minorities. 'Race', or ethnicity, needs to be considered because it is strongly related to an individual's life chances and opportunities (Rathwell and Phillips, 1986) – and these are major determinants of health. There is a considerable body of evidence that shows that 'ethnicity' is associated with health status (Nazroo, 1997). 'Ethnicity', which refers to variations in the human species created by the interplay of geography and heredity (Aslam *et al.*, 2001) is, however, notoriously difficult to measure because it is not clear what the best indicator of ethnicity should be. There is debate about how to define ethnicity and thereby measure it. Should it be one's self-assigned ethnic status? Should it be based on the country of birth? Should it be based on one's parents' country of birth? In practice a composite measure is often used. Consequently, when examining data on ethnicity and health it is important to take into account the precise way in which ethnicity has been defined. Tables 6.5

Table 6.5
Standardised
mortality ratios (SMR)
by country of birth for
men aged 20–64 years
in England and Wales,
1991–93 (reproduced
with permission from
Davey Smith *et al.*,
2000)

	All causes	Ischaemic heart disease	Stroke	Lung cancer	Other cancer	Accidents and injuries	Suicide
Total	100	100	100	100	100	100	100
Caribbean	89*	60*	169*	59*	89	121	59*
West/South Africa	126*	83	315*	71	133*	75	59*
East Africa	123*	160*	113	37*	77	86	75*
Indian sub-continent	107*	150*	163*	48*	65*	80*	73*
India	106*	140*	140*	43*	64*	97	109
Pakistan	102	163*	148*	45*	62*	68*	34*
Bangladesh	133*	184*	324*	92	74*	40*	27*
Scotland	129*	117*	111	146*	114*	177*	149*
Ireland	135*	121*	130*	157*	120*	189*	135*

*p < 0.05.

	All causes	Ischaemic heart disease	Stroke	Lung cancer	Other cancer	Accidents and injuries	Suicide
Total	100	100	100	100	100	100	100
Caribbean	104	100	178*	32*	87	103	49*
West/South Africa	142*	69	215*	69	120	–	102
East Africa	127*	130	110	29*	98	–	129
Indian sub-continent	99	175*	132*	34*	68	93	115
Scotland	127*	127*	131*	164*	106	201*	153*
Ireland	115*	129*	118*	143*	98	160*	144*

*p < 0.05.

Table 6.6
Standardised mortality ratios (SMR) by country of birth for women aged 20–64 years in England and Wales, 1991–93 (reproduced with permission from Davey Smith *et al.*, 2000)

and 6.6 show how mortality rates vary for both men and women amongst ethnic groups, where the country of birth is taken as the 'measure' of ethnicity.

The standardised mortality ratios (SMRs) for both men and women vary according to their country of birth for all causes of death (Tables 6.5, 6.6). For example, men who were born in Bangladesh, Ireland, Scotland and West/South Africa have higher levels of mortality for all causes of death. We can also see that there are variations between the causes of death. For example, whilst death rates from lung cancer are high for both men and women whose country of birth is Scotland or Ireland, comparable death rates from lung cancer are relatively low amongst those people who were born in the other countries listed in the tables. Ischaemic heart disease, by contrast, is a major cause of death amongst all groups with the exception of those born in West/South Africa. Moreover, the incidence of diabetes is very high amongst immigrants from the Indian sub-continent compared to other groups (Aslam et al., 2001).

Table 6.7 shows that amongst men and women aged 60 years and over, those from Pakistan and Bangladesh are more likely than their white counterparts to report that they have experienced poor health which restricted their activity in the previous two weeks. A number of explanations have been put forward in an attempt to make sense of such variations in health status between ethnic groups. Davey Smith and his colleagues (2000) have identified seven 'models of explanation' from the ongoing debates:

1. *Artefact explanations*. These draw attention to the processes involved in data collection and measurement. Indeed, as we have already noted, trying to collect data on 'ethnicity' is highly complex and it is likely that some data may, at the very worst, be spurious or misleading. However, the weight of evidence now is such that it is accepted that variations in health status and life-chances do exist between different ethnic groups.

	White (excluding Irish)	Irish	Indian	Pakistani, Bangladeshi	Black Caribbean	Chi square sign. P<
Men						
60–74	16	16	17	43	23	0.001
75 and over	18	24	2	–	3	–
All aged 60 and over	17	18	17	40	23	0.001
Women						
60–74	18	21	26	37	19	0.08
75 and over	24	25	4	1	9	0.06
All aged 60 and over	20	22	25	36	27	0.1
All						
60–74	17	19	21	41	21	0.001
75 and over	22	25	6	1	46	0.04
All aged 60 and over	19	20	21	39	25	0.001

Table 6.7 Percentage of persons aged 60 years and over reporting an illness or injury that restricted their activity in the previous two weeks, by age, sex and ethnicity, 1991–96, Great Britain (reproduced with permission from Evandrou, 2000)

2. *Migration*. It is suggested that the social processes associated with migration itself may contribute to the apparent differences in the health status of different groups. It may be that only the healthiest individuals tend to migrate, or conversely the experience of migration itself may be stressful and damaging to health. However, such explanations are likely to have limited impact upon people's health status over time and so can only form part of the story.

3. *Socio-economic factors* such as occupational class, income, housing tenure, etc. have been suggested as accounting for the differences. Certainly, some ethnic minorities, for example Bangladeshi, Pakistani and Caribbean groups, are over-represented in social classes IV and V and are more likely to be unemployed (Nazroo, 1997). Moreover, there are significant variations in terms of income between ethnic groups. For example, the mean income of Pakistani and Bangladeshi house-holds who are in social classes I and II is less than the mean income of white households who are classified as being in social classes IV and V (Davey Smith *et al.*, 2000). It is pur-ported, therefore, that it is not ethnicity *per se* that accounts for the differences in health but the socio-economic factors that are experienced by those in particular groupings.

4. *Culture, beliefs and behaviour* of different social groups. Most commonly invoked in these types of explanations are patterns of health-related behaviours such as smoking, drinking, diet, alcohol and exercise. So too are issues of child rearing and the organisation of family and kinship. It is, however, extremely difficult to disaggregate these factors, and evidence of associ-ations with health outcomes tends to be contradictory.

5. *Racism*. Potentially impacts on health status in a number of ways. It can do so indirectly in that racism may be the reason

why some ethnic groups experience socio-economic disadvantage. More direct impacts of racism may be racial harassment and discrimination which may induce poor health.

6. *Biological* reasons for the patterning of health. Genetic variations are sometimes cited as the reasons for differences in the prevalence of conditions such as diabetes and hypertension. It is important to recognise here that genetic factors, and indeed other physiological characteristics, are meshed within social and environmental factors.

7. *Health service access and use.* Proponents of these explanations point to the inequitable access to care, with people from ethnic groups being placed at a disadvantage. Certainly the routes to health care are complex and inequalities in the provision and use of health services are well documented (Acheson Report, 1998).

It is evident from these seven sets of explanations that the links between ethnic variations and health status are complex. It is unlikely that any one explanation could account for all the differences found in the data on ethnic variations and health. When assessing the merits and demerits of these explanations it is important to pay careful attention to the available empirical evidence. It is all too easy to conjecture on the basis of a particular data set, and to conclude that apparent differences between ethnic minority groups may be intrinsically associated with a given group's 'ethnicity' or 'race'. However, their genes, their culture, their behaviours cannot be divorced from other social, economic or political factors.

As we have discussed, Western society is unequal. This inequality manifests itself in lessened life and health chances on the basis of social class, gender and occupation. However, it is also pertinent to appreciate that it is not only an individual's position in society that influences their health – prejudice and discrimination within society may also be important factors for health status and the experience of health care.

SOCIAL CLASS AND HEALTH

The concept of social class

If we consider the distribution of disease in society, it is apparent that some diseases are more prevalent among some members of the community than others. Therefore, the distribution of disease cannot be considered a purely random event to which every individual is equally susceptible. Moreover, an individual's prospect of longevity, and the quality of their health in general, owes less to chance and more to a number of predetermined

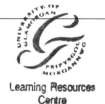

Learning Resources
Centre

factors. This discrepancy in the distribution of health and illness is particularly noticeable among the socially and economically disadvantaged.

One of the most easily identifiable and most frequently talked about inequalities which exists within British society is that of social class. Social class is regarded by some sociologists as the most fundamental system of social stratification within capitalist societies. The origins of class analysis can be traced back to the work of Karl Marx and Max Weber (see Chapter 1). Both sought to describe and explain the new class structure which emerged with the growth of industrial capitalism in early nineteenth-century Europe. Although their explanations of the origins and consequences of social class differed, they both believed class to be associated with economic circumstances. The origins, nature and implications of social class in the capitalist world are the subject of much debate within sociology. This need not unduly concern us here, but it is important to remember that social class, like all sociological concepts, is not static and unchanging but rather refers to a fluid or dynamic phenomenon. The eminent historian, E.P. Thompson (1977) illustrates this point with clarity in his work, *The Making of the English Working Class*:

'Sociologists who have stopped the time machine and, with a good deal of conceptual huffing and puffing, have gone down to the engine-room to look, tell us that nowhere at all have they been able to locate and classify a class. They can only find a multitude of people with different occupations, incomes, status-hierarchies, and the rest. Of course they are right, since class is not this or that part of the machine, but the way the machine works once it is set in motion – not this and that interest, but the friction of interests – the movement itself, the heat, the thundering noise. Class is a social and cultural formation (often finding institutional expression) which cannot be defined abstractly, or in isolation, but only in terms of relationships with other classes: and, ultimately, the definition can only be made in the medium of time – that is, action and reaction, change and conflict. When we speak of a class we are thinking of a very loosely defined body of people who share the same congeries of interests, social experiences, traditions and value-systems, who have a disposition to behave as a class, to define themselves in their actions and in their consciousness in relation to other groups of people in class ways. But class itself is not a thing, it is a happening.'

Social class classification

While gender and ethnicity are significant forms of stratification, social class has been used more extensively as an indicator of material circumstances. When we read a government document or hear reports of research findings that are related to social class, these are most likely to be based on one of two types of classifica-

	Social class	Examples of occupation
I	Professional	Doctor, lawyer, pharmacist
II	Intermediate	School teacher, manager, nurse
IIINM	Skilled non-manual	Secretary, shop assistant
IIIM	Skilled manual	Carpenter, electrician, cook
IV	Partly skilled	Postman, bus conductor, machine operator
V	Unskilled	Cleaner, labourer, dock worker

Table 6.8 The Registrar General's social class classification

tion that divide the population into a hierarchy of categories based on occupation. These are the Registrar General's social class classification and the Socio-Economic Group's classification which is used in the General Household Survey. These two classifications are similar, and for illustration the Registrar General's classification is reproduced in Table 6.8.

The limitations of social classification systems

Any classification system based simply on occupation has a number of shortcomings. To begin with these systems are based on a hierarchy of occupations that fail to take fully into account the continually changing nature of work patterns. For example, in recent years professional and managerial occupations have expanded rapidly, especially in the service or tertiary industries such as the financial, education and health sectors. There has also been a change in the nature of clerical work over the past fifty years. This change has not merely involved the introduction of technology into offices but has also resulted in an increased number of women recruited into this skilled, non-manual sector.

The classifications in terms of occupation may be misleading, as women in non-manual occupations, which are classified as higher than manual work, may well receive lower pay than male manual workers, or be employed on a part-time basis. Clearly, occupational categories fail to take into account those people who are not working or, more accurately, those who are not economically active such as the unemployed, retired, some people with disabilities, and women who work at home. Further, when classifying families, only the occupation of the head of the household is taken into account. This may not accurately reflect the household in which other members may add significantly to the overall income. When classifying families on the basis of the occupation of the head of the household there is also an assumption that the income and the associated resources are distributed equitably within the family. However, in practice this has been shown not to be the case – for example, a resource such as the 'family car' frequently used by the husband was found to be rarely available to the wife on a daily basis (Graham, 1984).

Despite these shortcomings, and in the absence of more sensitive measures, occupational categories provide an appropriate means of collating data which can be related to people's socio-economic circumstances. Consequently, we shall consider how these socio-economic indicators can be related to health status.

Social class and health: the evidence

The significance of social class in relation to health is that it is an indicator of material resources, i.e. income, wealth, material possessions and lifestyle. Indeed the *Report of the Working Group on Inequalities in Health*, which was submitted to the Secretary of State for Health in 1980, defined social class as:

'segments of the population sharing broadly similar styles of living and (for some sociologists) some shared perception of their collective condition' (Townsend and Davidson, 1982).

This report, widely referred to as the *Black Report* (after its chairman Sir Douglas Black), provided extensive evidence of inequalities in health status and of the use, availability and provision of health services between different social groups. The findings and recommendations of the *Black Report* resulted in a great deal of controversy at the time. In his response to the Report, the Health Secretary, Patrick Jenkin, noted that, *'It will come as a disappointment to many that over long periods since the inception of the NHS there is generally little sign of health inequalities in Britain actually diminishing and, in some cases increasing.'* However, he felt that the proposals which he claimed would cost upwards of £2 billion a year were 'unrealistic'; he therefore would make no commitment to a change in existing health policy. *The Health Divide: Inequalities in the 1980s*, published in 1987 (Whitehead, 1987), examined how the picture had changed since the *Black Report*, and considered what progress, if any, had been made towards implementing the recommendations of the 1980 Working Group. It emerged that for most areas of health the social class inequalities remained. We are now in the twenty-first century and such inequalities remain. The *Independent Inquiry into Inequalities in Health* – the 'Acheson Report' (1998) found that inequalities in health had in fact widened since the publication of the *Black Report*, and this was largely due to the growing gap between the rich and poor within the UK.

Over this period, the life expectancy of men and women has increased. In 1981 a man's life expectancy was 70.9 years and a woman's was 76.8 years; by 1998 these had increased to 74.9 and 79.8 years respectively (Office of National Statistics, 2001). However, life expectancy varies between social classes to such an extent that the life expectancy for men and women in the lower social classes today approximates overall life expectancies in the

| | Women (35–64) | | | Men (35–64) | | |
	1976–81	1981–85	1986–92	1976–81	1981–85	1986–92
All causes						
I/II	338	344	270	621	539	455
III (non-manual)	371	387	305	860	658	484
III (manual)	467	396	356	802	691	624
IV/V	508	445	418	951	824	764
Ratio IV/V–I/II	1.50	1.29	1.55	1.53	1.53	1.68

Table 6.9 Age standardised mortality rates per 100,000 people, by social class for men and women aged 35–64 in England and Wales, 1976–92 (reproduced with permission from the Acheson Report, 1998)

Table 6.10 Perinatal and infant mortality rates per 1,000 births (within marriage only) by social class 1978/79 and 1999 (Howard *et al.*, 2001; reproduced with kind permission of the Child Poverty Action Group)

late 1970s and early 1980s. In fact, in the UK the life expectancy differences between social class I and V is 5.2 years for men and 3.4 years for women (Pantazis and Gordon, 2000). The Acheson Report (1998) presented extensive data showing the growing difference in mortality rates across the social spectrum for many of the major causes of death, including coronary heart disease, lung cancer, respiratory disease, strokes and suicide. The summary statistics for all causes of death are shown in Table 6.9.

A striking example of the extent to which social class correlates with inequalities in health status is apparent from the statistics on rates of perinatal and infant mortality. Table 6.10 shows that infant mortality (i.e. death within the first year of life) inside marriage was almost twice as high in social classes IV than in social classes I and II. A similar class gradient is evident for perinatal mortality (death within the first week of life). Women who are categorised as belonging to social classes I and II have the lowest rates of infant mortality. Thus, it is apparent that the rates both of stillbirths and of infant mortality are related to a person's social grouping. Further, it is clear from Table 6.10 that whilst the overall mortality rates have decreased, the ratios between the social classes have increased.

Linked with inequalities in health between social groupings, there are also marked differences in life expectancy according to the geographical location in which people live (Table 6.11). Moreover, within these regions there may also be marked differences in life expectancy. For example, a study in Sheffield found that there

| Social class | Perinatal | | Infant | |
	1978/79	1999	1978/79	1999
I	11.9	5.8	9.8	3.8
II	12.3	6.2	10.1	3.8
III (non-manual)	13.9	8.2	11.1	5.0
III (manual)	15.1	7.7	12.4	5.1
IV	16.7	9.9	13.6	6.5
V	20.3	11.0	17.2	8.4
Other	20.4	9.7	23.3	7.3
Ratio class V:I	1.71	1.89	1.8	2.21

	All causes
Males	
United Kingdom	969
Northern and Yorkshire	1,039
North West	1,060
Trent	982
West Midlands	980
Anglia and Oxford	879
North Thames	912
South Thames	885
South and West	859
England	947
Wales	973
Scotland	1,132
Northern Ireland	1,017
Females	
United Kingdom	1,045
Northern and Yorkshire	1,117
North West	1,149
Trent	1,060
West Midlands	1,045
Anglia and Oxford	989
North Thames	971
South Thames	962
South and West	932
England	1,025
Wales	1,057
Scotland	1,207
Northern Ireland	1,052
All persons	
United Kingdom	1,014
Northern and Yorkshire	1,084
North West	1,108
Trent	1,031
West Midlands	1,021
Anglia and Oxford	946
North Thames	950
South Thames	929
South and West	904
England	994
Wales	1,022
Scotland	1,170
Northern Ireland	1,037

*Rates standardised to the mid-1991 United Kingdom population for males and females separately.

Table 6.11 Age adjusted mortality rates* per 100,000 population, by region and gender, 1998 (reproduced with permission from the Office of National Statistics, 2000)

was a difference in life expectancy of almost eight years between the most affluent and the most deprived areas within the city (Thunhurst, 1985). This may be the outcome of factors such as people's occupations, their housing conditions and their exposure to environmental hazards such as road traffic, pollution and availability of safe play areas for children.

Unemployment and health

Whilst certain occupations can result in detrimental effects on an individual's health, so too can being out of work. Fagin (1984) in his report *The Forsaken Families: The Effects of Unemployment on Family Life* documented the extent to which financial worries, resulting from unemployment, had an impact on family tension. This tension was manifested in high rates of depression, asthma or headaches in all the family members. Similarly, a longitudinal study of twenty-six shipyard workers and their families found that men who had been made redundant, experienced depressive reactions, in spite of good financial compensation (Joelson and Wahlquist, 1987). A central theme to their findings was that when a person lost their job they also felt they had lost their identity. Their previously structured lives had been disrupted, so that for example: *'work ... regulates strain and rest and the time spent with one's family and away from it'*. Work was also seen as evidence of the men's competence and knowledge. Whilst at work, the men had clearly defined relations with other workers and with their workmates. On being made redundant, most of the single men lost the majority of their social contacts.

Further evidence that people who are unemployed tend to have poorer health than those who are in employment has been provided by Maclure and Stewart (1984) who found that 28 per cent of unemployed men reported long-standing illness, compared with 25 per cent of working men. Children of the unemployed were also found to be more prone to poor health. Data from the 1981 census were used to show that children living in deprived districts of Glasgow were more likely to be admitted to hospital than children in non-deprived districts. Unemployment has also been found to be associated with higher levels of suicide, and has been an important factor contributing to the increased rate of suicide in the UK (Lewis and Sloggett, 1998).

We have provided only a brief introduction to the extensive literature on the relationship between social class and health. However, from the studies in this area it is clearly evident that:

1. Inequalities in health apply at every stage of life, from birth throughout adult life to old age.
2. All the major killer diseases affect the poor more than the affluent.
3. Chronic sickness is more prevalent in less-favoured occupations.
4. The unemployed and their families have been found to experience poor mental and physical health.

Social class and health: the explanations

As we have illustrated, there are extensive data suggesting the existence of a correlation between social class and health status. However, evidence of a statistical correlation does not of itself provide us with an adequate explanation for these inequalities. The data provide only the starting point. Presented with such evidence we need to try and make sense of it and search for appropriate explanations. In other words, we have seen that there is a relationship between the two variables: social class and health. However, this relationship requires further explanation because we cannot be sure which is the causal variable simply by presenting the data. Methodologically, then, we need to identify which is the independent and which is the dependent variable. That is to say, does social class determine health or does health determine social class?

Some sociologists have argued that the reason for the inequalities in health is that people who experience poor health tend to move down the occupational scale. These sociologists regard a person's social class position as being dependent on their health (Goldberg and Morrison, 1963; Illsley, 1986). Wadsworth (1986) for example, using data from the National Survey of Health and Development Cohort Study, showed how a series of illnesses in childhood could affect social mobility. Boys who were seriously ill were more likely than others to experience a fall in occupational class by the time they were 26 years old, although others have argued that overall this effect is of a very minor nature (Blane, 1985). Conversely, it has been argued that health is dependent on an individual's socio-economic circumstances, i.e. their occupation, financial resources and standard of living. One variant of this perspective maintains that people from lower socio-economic groups may be less inclined to protect their future health and tend, from an early age, to adopt lifestyles that are potentially harmful. Another orientation of the view that health is the outcome of social class is that the material and environmental conditions in which people live directly impinge on their health. This argument then suggests that poor health may be attributed less to the individual and more to the individual's physical and social environment.

Both the *Black Report* and the *Health Divide* assessed the validity of the explanations which have formed the main strands of the debate concerning social class and health in recent decades. They have identified four explanations for the link between the two. The explanations are summarised by Sally Macintyre in Table 6.12, and are categorised into 'hard' and soft' versions of the explanations.

Explanation	'Hard' version	'Soft' version
Artefact	No relation between class and mortality; purely an artefact of measurement	Magnitude of observed class gradients will depend on the measurement of both class and health
Natural/social selection	Health determines class position, therefore class gradients are morally neutral and explained 'away'	Health can contribute to achieved class position and help to explain observed gradients
Materialist/structural	Material, physical conditions of life associated with the class structure are the complete explanation for class gradients in health	Physical and psycho-social features associated with the class structure influence health and contribute to observed gradients
Cultural/behavioural	Health-damaging behaviours freely chosen by individuals in different social classes explain away social class gradients	Health-damaging behaviours are differentially distributed across social classes and contribute to observed gradients

Table 6.12 The two versions of explanations of health inequalities (reproduced with permission from Macintyre, 1997)

The artefact explanation

The artefact explanation proposes that health inequalities are artificial rather than real. They are merely a function of inadequate tools of measurement. That is to say, the 'tools' or 'indicators' used to establish a link between social class and health were not sufficiently sensitive for what they were intended to measure. The quality and reproducibility of the data however would seem to refute this argument.

The social selection explanation

The social selection explanation presents the case that we have outlined above; namely, that health determines social class. The finding that health inequalities are related to social status is a consequence of the notion that those with good health tend to improve their social position, while those in poor health 'drift' downwards.

The cultural/behavioural explanation

Cultural/behavioural arguments claim that certain patterns of behaviour – for instance, smoking, lack of exercise and excessive consumption of alcohol – are more prevalent amongst certain groups in society than others. This explanation assumes that the individual is able to overcome societal and environmental pressures to commence or continue these patterns of behaviour if they so desire.

The materialist or structuralist explanation

The materialist or structuralist postulate emphasises the circumstances in which people live. From this point of view, poor health becomes the outcome of material deprivation. Whilst, for example, nutrition may be an important etiological factor in ill-health, the focus is on factors that influence a person's ability to make choices about the food they buy. It has been calculated that a healthy diet, as defined in the National Advisory Council on Nutrition Education report, could cost up to 35 per cent more than the typical diet of a low income family (Whitehead, 1987). Furthermore, there is evidence that poor people pay proportionately more for their food because they have to buy 'little and often' from local shops which are more expensive than larger outlets. This is because they do not have the resources to buy in bulk, nor do they have transport to access out-of-town shopping facilities (Howard *et al.*, 2001).

The *Black Report* found, in the light of the extensive evidence the working group had considered, that the materialist explanation of health inequalities was the most viable. Subsequently the *Health Divide* found:

'Fresh evidence [which] shows that life-style and material living conditions influence health and vary with occupational class. Furthermore, recent in-depth studies have increased understanding of how living and working conditions impose severe restrictions on an individual's ability to choose a healthy life style. They have provided fresh insight into the way behaviours are influenced by social conditions and argue for a policy which recognises the link between the two, in preference to policies which focus solely on the individual' (Whitehead, 1987).

This explanation has also been endorsed by the Acheson Report (1998), and the current government has stated that a central thrust of its policies is to create a *'fairer society'* and wants to tackle the *'causes of poverty and social exclusion, not just to alleviate the symptoms'* (Department of Health, 1999). The extent to which this aim will be met remains to be seen, but the New Labour government has prioritised child poverty and introduced fiscal measures such as the Working Family Tax Credit to overcome it. Poverty and inequality, however, are so endemic in contemporary society, much work remains to be done.

PSYCHO-SOCIAL CIRCUMSTANCES AND HEALTH

The association between occupation or social group and health chances has been explored by Marmott and Theorell (1988). They have reviewed the evidence that psycho-social work conditions influence the risk factors associated with coronary heart disease. Those workers who had least skill and least discretion or authority over decisions, or who lacked social support at work, were found to be most likely to experience stress and adopt unhealthy behaviour such as smoking. Hence, while the relationship between heart disease and stress and smoking has been established, this may not constitute an adequate explanation of a person's ill-health because there are often other factors associated with their social circumstances which should be taken into account. It has been suggested that it may be something about the way our society is organised, and how it is experienced, which accounts for differences in health outcomes, rather than individual behaviours. This suggestion forms the basis of what has come to be known as the 'Wilkinson hypothesis'. The researcher Richard Wilkinson (1996) has argued that societies that are more unequal are less healthy than those that are more egalitarian. According to his view inequality *per se* is bad for people's health. Unequal societies are less cohesive and more socially divisive. This, he suggests, is because people have less control over their circumstances, are socially isolated, and may have limited forms of social support. This is referred to as the psycho-social explanation for health inequalities because it draws attention to the psychological impacts of social structures. Wilkinson suggests that:

'The social consequences of people's differing circumstances in terms of stress, self esteem and social relations, may now be one of the most important influences on health' (Wilkinson, 1992).

The idea that social cohesion and integration is good for health was demonstrated empirically by the sociologist Émile Durkheim in the nineteenth century (see Chapter 1). He found that suicide rates were lower in those countries which had higher levels of social integration. This Durkheimian idea is evident in the work of many influential writers of the contemporary period. In particular, Wilkinson is impressed by the work of Putnam, an American political scientist, who developed the notion of 'social capital'. Social capital refers to the degree of trust, integration and cohesion within a society or a community. The New Labour government has also been impressed by this American academic, and this is evident in their policies which are designed to tackle social exclusion and foster communities. Examples range from the Urban Regeneration Programme to Health Action Zones which encourage disparate organisations and agencies to work together to improve all aspects of the lives of people living within deprived areas. The Wilkinson thesis, and indeed Putnam's notion of social capital, as well as influencing policy has generated much debate. For example, there is a view that attempts to improve poor areas will not tackle the more fundamental issue of inequalities unless the gap between the rich and poor is narrowed and income is redistributed.

How evidence regarding inequalities and health is interpreted has important implications for health policy and for decision-making in terms of the allocation of financial resources and the types of provision for health required. Like the findings of the epidemiologists we described earlier in this chapter, it would seem that any real attempt to improve health lies beyond health care as it has been traditionally conceived and must address wider social issues.

Summary

- Health chances are determined by social factors, including gender, ethnicity, social class and employment status
- Social class is a widely used indicator of material resources
- Four broad explanations have been identified for the link between health and social class: the artefact, the social selection, the cultural/behavioural and the materialist explanations
- Social cohesion and integration are beneficial for health.

Further reading

Acheson Report (1998) *Independent Inquiry into Inequalities in Health*, London, Stationery Office.

Graham, G. (2000) *Understanding Health Inequalities*, Buckingham, Open University Press.

Pantazis, C. and Gordon, D. (2000) *Tackling Inequalities: Where Are We Now and What Can Be Done?*, Bristol, The Policy Press.

Wilkinson, R. (1996) *Unhealthy Societies: the Afflictions of Inequality*, London, Routledge.

References

Acheson Report (1998) *Independent Inquiry into Inequalities in Health*, London, Stationery Office.

Arber, S. and Thomas, H. (2001) From women's health to gender analysis of health. In: W.C. Cockerham (ed.) *The Blackwell Companion to Medical Sociology*, Oxford, Blackwell, pp. 94–113.

Aslam, M., Jessa, F. and Wilson, J. (2001) Ethnic minorities. In: K.M.G. Taylor and G. Harding (eds) *Pharmacy Practice*, London, Taylor and Francis, pp. 273–287.

Blane, D. (1985) An assessment of the Black Report's explanation of health inequalities. *Sociology of Health and Illness*, 7, 423–445.

Crompton, R. (1997) *Women and Work in Modern Britain*, Oxford, Oxford University Press.

Davey Smith, L., Chaturvedi, N., Harding, S. and Nazroo, J. (2000) Ethnic inequalities in health: a review of the epidemiological evidence. *Critical Public Health*, 10, 375–408.

Department of Health (1999) *Reducing Health Inequalities: An Action Report*, London, Department of Health.

Evandrou, M. (2000) Ethnic inequalities in health in later life. *Health Statistics Quarterly*, 8, 20–28.

Evans, M. (1998) Social security: dismantling the pyramids? In: H. Glennerster and J. Hills (eds) *The State of Welfare: The Economics of Social Spending*, Oxford, Oxford University Press.

Fagin, L. (1984) *The Forsaken Families: The Effects of Unemployment on Family Life*, Harmondsworth, Penguin.

Goldberg, E.M. and Morrison, S.L. (1963) Schizophrenia and social class. *British Journal of Psychiatry*, 109, 785–802.

Graham, H. (1984) *Women, Health and the Family*, Brighton, Wheatsheaf Books.

Howard, M., Garnham, A., Fimister, G. and Veit-Wilson, J. (2001) *Poverty: The Facts*, London, Child Poverty Action Group.

Illsley, R. (1986) Occupational class selection and the production of inequalities in health. *Quarterly Journal of Social Affairs*, 2, 151–165.

Joelson, L. and Wahlquist, L. (1987) The psychological meaning of job insecurity and job loss: results of a longitudinal study. *Social Science and Medicine*, 25, 179–182.

Lahelma, E., Arber, S., Martikainen, P., Rahkonen, O. and Silventoinen, K. (2001) The myth of gender differences in health: social structural determinants across adult ages in Britain and Finland. *Current Sociology*, 49, pp. 31–54.

Lewis, G. and Sloggett, A. (1998) Suicide, deprivation, and unemployment: record linkage study. *British Medical Journal*, 317, 1283–1286.

Macintyre, S. (1997) The Black Report and beyond: what are the issues? *Social Science and Medicine*, 48, 89–98.

Macintyre, S., Hunt, K. and Sweeting, H. (1996) Gender differences in health: are things really as simple as they seem? *Social Science and Medicine*, 42, 617–624.

Maclure, A. and Stewart, G.T. (1984) Admissions of children to hospital in Glasgow: relation to unemployment and other deprivation variables. *Lancet*, ii, 682–688.

Marmott, M. and Theorell, T. (1988) Social class and cardio-vascular disease: the contribution of work. *International Journal of Health Services*, 18, 659–674.

Miller, J. and Glendinning, C. (1992) It all really starts in the family home: gender and poverty. In: C. Glendinning and J. Miller (eds) *Women and Poverty in Britain in the 1990s*, Hemel Hempstead, Harvester Wheatsheaf, pp. 3–10.

Nazroo, J.Y. (1997) *The Health of Britain's Ethnic Minorities: Findings From a National Survey*, London, Policy Studies Institute.

Office of National Statistics (1988) *Social Trends*, London, HMSO.

Office of National Statistics (2000*) Living in Britain: Results from the General Household Survey*, London, Office of National Statistics.

Office of National Statistics (2001) *Social Trends 31*, London, HMSO.

Pantazis, C. and Gordon, D. (2000) *Tackling Inequalities: Where Are We Now and What Can Be Done?*, Bristol, The Policy Press.

Rainford, L., Mason, V., Hickman, M. and Morgan, A. (1998) *Health in England 1998: Investigating the Links Between Social Inequalities and Health*. London, Stationery Office.

Rathwell, T. and Phillips, D. (eds) (1986) *Health, Race and Ethnicity*, London, Croom Helm.

Thompson, E.P. (1977) *The Making of the English Working Class*, London, Penguin.

Thunhurst, C. (1985) *Poverty and Health in the City of Sheffield*, Sheffield, Environmental Health Dept, Sheffield City Council.

Townsend, P. and Davidson, N. (1982) *Inequalities in Health: The Black Report*, Harmondsworth, Penguin.

Wadsworth, M.E.J. (1986) Serious illness in childhood and its association with later life achievements. In: R.G. Wilkinson (ed.) *Class and Health: Research and Longitudinal Data*, London, Tavistock.

Whitehead, M. (1987) *The Health Divide: Inequalities in the 1980s*, London, Health Education Council.

Wilkinson, R. (1992) Income distribution and life expectancy. *British Medical Journal*, 304, 165–168.

Wilkinson, R. (1996) *Unhealthy Societies: the Afflictions of Inequality*, London, Routledge.

7 The Occupational Status of Pharmacy

INTRODUCTION

In analysing the occupational status of pharmacy, and whether or not pharmacy should be considered a profession, it is first necessary to explore exactly what is meant by the term 'profession'. This chapter aims to offer such an analysis. When reading this chapter, it will be beneficial to reflect upon what it means to be a pharmacist, what it means to be a health professional, the position of pharmacists within the community and their relationship with other health workers.

There is an extensive literature on the sociology of the professions and considerable debate over what actually constitutes a profession. There are, however, certain attributes of an occupation which have generally come to be accepted as distinguishing it as a profession. Some occupations, in particular those of Law and Medicine, have acquired a pre-eminent status in society, becoming institutions with considerable prestige and power. This distinguishes them from other occupations. For these occupations, the term 'professional' has an important sociological meaning, one that is different from its more colloquial sense. For example, when we speak of professional footballers we imply that they are skilled and are paid to play their chosen sport. However, they do not possess the key characteristics that define a profession in the sociological sense. Let us look, then, at the features that define a profession and then turn to consider whether or not pharmacy can be considered a profession.

SOCIOLOGICAL APPROACHES TO PROFESSIONALISATION

The question as to why some occupations rise to the status of profession whilst others do not is a sociological puzzle which calls for an explanation. Since Parsons (1939) published his seminal paper, 'The professions and the social structure', many theories have been postulated. Until the 1970s, most writers tried to explain the professions' unique position in society by way of definitions. That is, they tried to identify or define those characteristics of an occupation which were special or peculiar to professional status. This resulted in a proliferation of literature that listed the particular attributes of a profession – for example, Goode (1960). This has been referred to as the 'attribute' or 'trait' approach. The traits outlined in Box 7.1 are those most frequently cited.

Rather than attempting to simply define the attributes of professions, some sociologists have suggested that professions have achieved their importance or status because they perform functions which are vital to the workings of modern industrialised society. Sociologists refer to this as the 'structuralist–functionalist explanation'. A structuralist–functionalist perspective views society as analogous to an organism in which all the parts function in a way that ensures the continued well-being of the whole organism, rather like the various physiological systems of the human body. All social institutions have a use, otherwise they would cease to have a function and would quickly disappear. Complex industrial societies need expert knowledge, and professions perform the function of applying their expert knowledge for the benefit of the community. Whilst both the trait and functionalist approaches have since been surpassed by more critical and realistic analyses, we can say that professions:

- possess certain core characteristics or traits
- fulfil important societal functions

Core characteristics of a profession

Certain 'core' characteristics have been identified that are possessed by all professions. These are summarised in Box 7.2.

To become accepted into a profession, an individual must undergo a period of training. This is invariably long (for example, usually seven years for architecture and five years for medicine) and highly specialised. This high degree of training is required, since in order to practice the professional must possess a specialised knowledge which is not readily accessible to the rest of

Box 7.2 The core characteristics of a profession	• Specialised knowledge and lengthy training • Service orientation • Monopoly of practice • Self-regulation

the population. In many ways it is this specialised knowledge that sets professionals apart from the consumers of their services, who do not possess such knowledge or expertise. Consequently, they are reliant on the 'expert's' service. Indeed, a second characteristic of a profession is service orientation. This means that professionals should work in the best interests of their clients, and should not be intent on pursuing their own self-interest. This characteristic is very important because a profession has a monopoly of practice in their given field. This monopoly is granted and secured by the State. In other words, it is illegal for people other than members of the profession to carry out defined tasks; for example, it is illegal for anyone other than a qualified surgeon to carry out a heart transplant.

In addition to the restriction of practice, a profession monitors or 'polices' itself. Friedson (1970a) argues that a profession is *distinct from other occupations in that it has been given the right to control its own work*. A profession regulates the system of training, decides who is eligible to enter the profession and assesses who is competent to practice within the profession. That is to say, they 'self-regulate'. Professionals maintain that the unusual degree of skill and knowledge involved in professional activities means that non-professionals are not properly equipped to evaluate or regulate the professions' activities. If a professional does not perform competently or ethically, his or her peers preside over the outcome; they are constituted as a professional regulatory body. In the case of pharmacy, this is the Royal Pharmaceutical Society of Great Britain.

It is often claimed that professions as social institutions wield power and influence, in that to a great extent most legislation that affects a profession is shaped by that profession itself. The 'restrictive practices' of all the professions are constantly under review and through the introduction of certain mechanisms they are becoming more accountable to external agencies. An example of this is the National Health Service (General Medical and Pharmaceutical Services) Amendment Regulations (1985), known as the 'Limited List', which restricted the medicinal products of a particular class, such as cough remedies and benzodiazepines, that the NHS would pay for if prescribed. This amendment was attacked at the time of its introduction by both the pharmaceutical industry and the medical profession as an encroachment on clinical judgement and a curtailment of the clinical freedom of general practitioners. More recently, the establishment of the National Institute of Clinical Excellence (NICE) as a Special Health Authority for England and Wales in 1999 to appraise the efficacy of new and existing treatments, and issue guidelines to practitioners, introduced a framework for decision-making in clinical medicine. This policy initiative is an example of what is termed evidence-based health care, which is the attempt to ensure that clinical and professional practice is guided and informed by systematic research. In other words, professional decisions and actions should not just be based on the individual knowledge and expertise of practitioners but instead on scientific assessments of effectiveness (see Chapter 5).

Also impacting on the autonomous functioning of health professions has been the response to emergent evidence of malpractice and poor self-regulation among the professions, in particular medicine. Self-regulation of professionals has come under the scrutiny of the government, which has sought to increase the public accountability of the regulatory mechanisms operated by the health professions, including pharmacy.

Professional judgement

The notion of professional judgment is central to any discussion of professions. This is because, in order to remain exclusive to the members of the profession itself, its work must not become routinised or rationalised. Professionals have, as a result of their training, acquired the ability to make assessments or judgements on the basis of experience and skill. Jamous and Peloille (1970) have described this in terms of the 'I/T' ratio; that is, the profession has claims to greater indeterminate knowledge (I) than technical knowledge (T). Indeterminate knowledge is personal knowledge and personal judgement, whilst technical knowledge refers to knowledge that is rational and codified.

Freidson (1970b), in his book *Professional Dominance*, termed this the *'clinical mentality'*. He distinguished the medical practitioner (the clinician) from the scientist or theorist. The clinician's primary orientation is towards action, to an extent that he or she may prefer to do something with very uncertain chances of success, than do nothing at all. The practitioner, Freidson argues, *'believes what he is doing'*; that is, professionals are likely to display personal commitment to their chosen course of action. The practitioner is essentially a pragmatist, relying on results rather than theory, trusting personal rather than book knowledge. It may be pertinent, in this light, to consider whether pharmacists are clinicians or scientists.

The paramedical professions, for example nursing and physiotherapy, are in a different position to the medical profession, for while it is legitimate for them to take orders from, and be assessed by, physicians, it is not legitimate for them to give orders or evaluate the work of doctors. Hence, while they possess many of the attributes of a profession, in that there is a system of registration and licensing, and formal standards of training together with regulation of their own members, they do not enjoy the full autonomy of a profession. On this basis, some would regard these as 'incomplete professions'.

The process of professionalisation

We have so far assumed that what constitutes a profession is dependent on something special or superior about a particular occupation; its possession of knowledge and skills that ensures total control over a particular sphere of work. However, whilst the length of training, service orientation, code of ethics and expertise are all significant in persuading the State and the public of their importance, they are not 'causes' of an occupation achieving professional status nor, it would seem, are they objectively determined attributes. Wright (1979), in his paper 'A study of the legitimisation of knowledge: the success of medicine and the failure of astrology', has illustrated this point. He argues that the success of medicine as a profession does not result from anything intrinsic in medical knowledge. Indeed, when physicians first began to organise themselves into groups there was no evidence that their knowledge and methods were any more effective than those of astrologists. The differences lay rather in the social position of doctors, the social position of their clients and, ultimately, their success in legitimising their activities.

This sociological perspective, then, views the process of professionalisation as one of occupational control. Professional autonomy is seen to be the outcome of the interaction between political and economic powers, and occupational representation, which is often helped by educational institutions that persuade the State that the occupation's work is reliable and valuable. That is to say, occupations achieve their status as professions as the result of political struggles and power conflicts between different interest groups. An occupation becomes a profession, not so much because of improvements in its skills and knowledge but rather because the profession's leaders are successful in convincing the State that autonomy and self-regulation are desirable. It may then not be the characteristics of professionals *per se* that determine their status so much as *their* relationships with the State, clients, and other occupations.

Johnson (1989) developed this perspective in his book, *Professions and Power*. Johnson rejects the 'trait' theory of professionalism as inadequate. Instead of pondering the question as to whether an occupation is a profession, it may be more appropriate to consider the circumstances in which individuals attempt to turn an occupation into a profession. It has been suggested that:

'This line of approach avoids many of the pitfalls opened up by frankly evaluating definitions of the professions. It concentrates upon determining circumstances under which occupational groups make an avowal of professionalism and leaves to others the task of judging how close they come to living up to the professional' (King, 1968, quoted by Johnson, 1989).

How successful an occupation's claim to professionalism is depends in part on the power relationship between the occupation's members and those served by them. An important element of this relationship, Johnson observes, is that of 'mystification'. Members of an occupation which aspires to professional status may only achieve their aim in circumstances whereby they are able successfully to promote their services as esoteric. In creating a dependence upon their skills, members of such occupations reduce the areas of knowledge and experience they have in common with those they serve. This increase in the 'social distance' between themselves and their clients provides professionals with an opportunity for autonomous control over their practices. In other words, by promoting the esoteric nature of their services, professionals ward off potential challenges to their status from the lay public. Hence, it is not simply a list of attributes that defines a profession; rather it is the public's willingness to accept, or their inability to successfully challenge, the professionals' area of expertise.

SOCIOLOGICAL PERSPECTIVES ON PHARMACY

The emergence of pharmacy

The preparation of medicines has occurred throughout history. The earliest records date from the second millennium BC, and this practice occurred in the ancient civilisations of Egypt, Babylonia, Asia, Greece and Rome. In Britain, during the Middle Ages, people having similar business interests or crafts grouped themselves together into Craft or Merchant Guilds. In the fourteenth century, the Company of Grocers of London was formed, of which apothecaries formed a sub-group. Two centuries later, the Society of Apothecaries was founded, and a subsequent Royal Charter established the apothecaries' monopoly in the dispensing of medicines against physicians' prescriptions, whilst members of the Company of Grocers retained the right to sell drugs and spices and later became known as 'druggists'. During the sixteenth century, people who were unable to either reach or afford a physician went to an apothecary for diagnosis, advice and supply of medicines.

Dispensing within the dispensary established by the College of Physicians in 1696 was carried out by assistants who were either druggists or apothecary's apprentices. These later became known as 'dispensing chemists'. Thus by the eighteenth century three rival groups were involved in the compounding and dispensing of medicines – namely, the apothecaries, druggists and dispensing chemists. In 1841 the Pharmaceutical Society of Great Britain was founded and incorporated by Royal Charter in 1843. The Society was founded to represent the interests of chemists and druggists, to raise their profile amongst the professions and to promote education and training. The Pharmacy Acts (1852 and 1868) restricted titles such as 'Pharmaceutical Chemist' and 'Pharmacist' to those registered with the Pharmaceutical Society, although membership was optional.

Since the Pharmacy and Poisons Act (1933), membership of the Pharmaceutical Society, together with the registration of premises, has been required for all persons engaged in the selling or dispensing of listed poisons and controlled medicines. The premises should at all times be under the personal supervision of a pharmacist. In 1988 the Pharmaceutical Society was renamed the Royal Pharmaceutical Society. More recent developments in the practice of pharmacy are outlined in Chapter 2. For a more detailed description and analysis of the development of pharmacy as an occupation readers are referred to Holloway (1991) and Anderson (2001).

Pharmacy as a profession

Pharmacy as an occupation possesses a number of characteristics of a profession as defined by the 'trait' theory:

1. *Monopoly of practice*. Currently, membership of the Royal Pharmaceutical Society is restricted to persons registered as Pharmaceutical Chemists under the terms of the Pharmacy Act, 1954. This act restricts entry to the Register of Pharmaceutical Chemists to those who have attained a degree in pharmacy at an approved School of Pharmacy, or who have passed the Pharmaceutical Chemist Qualifying Examination, provided they have paid the necessary fees and have completed, subsequent to passing a final degree examination, not less than one year of pre-registration training in an approved establishment. Additionally, in recent years, prior to registration, pharmacists have been required to pass a registration examination. Thus, since 1954, pharmacists have had, with very few exceptions, a State-legitimised monopoly over compounding and dispensing drugs. In addition, pharmacists have a monopoly over the sale of a particular legal class of medicines: Pharmacy Medicines.
2. *Specialised knowledge and lengthy training*. The undergraduate pharmacy degree course lasts four years and is followed (unless incorporated into a university 'sandwich' programme) by one year of pre-registration training and a registration examination. Upon successful completion of this extensive period of training pharmacists have unique knowledge and skills relating to the preparation, supply and therapeutic aspects of medicines use.
3. *Service-orientation*. Pharmacists provide a range of pharmaceutical services, including the dispensing of medicines and appli-

ances, treatment of minor ailments, and the provision of health care advice. Recently, the concepts of pharmaceutical care and medicines management have been introduced to encompass this range of services and highlight pharmacists' direct responsibility and accountability to patients for the outcomes of drug therapy.

4. *Self-regulation*. The Pharmacy and Poisons Act (1933) created the Statutory Committee of the Pharmaceutical Society. This Committee comprising mainly pharmacists and, under a chairperson *'having practical, legal experience'*, appointed by the Privy Council, acts as the disciplinary body for members of the pharmacy profession.

Thus, application of the 'trait' approach would seem to indicate that pharmacy may indeed be considered a profession. However, it is a matter of debate as to whether or not the full autonomy of pharmacy as a profession has been achieved (Shuval, 1981; Turner, 1995) and consequently some have argued that pharmacy is an incomplete profession (Denzin and Mettlin, 1968).

Five factors may be considered as hindering the professional autonomy of the pharmacist (Box 7.3).

Box 7.3 Factors hindering the professional autonomy of pharmacists

- Commercial arena in which pharmacy is practised
- Consumerism
- Corporatisation of pharmacy
- Increasing dependence on technology
- Dependence on physicians

1. Commercial arena in which pharmacy is practised
The large majority of pharmacists practice in the community (see Chapter 2). The commercial interests guiding a successful business (i.e. the maximisation of profit) may seem to be at odds with the ethos of impartial service orientation and professional altruism. Pharmacists practice both as 'impartial professionals' and business people, whether self-employed or as employees. This tension can result in pharmacists experiencing 'role ambiguity' or 'role strain' as they attempt to reconcile these duel facets. It raises the question as to whether the public view pharmacists as 'professionals' or shop-workers, since, as stated above, an occupation's relationship with the public is key to its privileged occupational standing. That said, some commentators have argued that professional altruism and commercial interests need not necessarily be in conflict (Dingwall and Wilson, 1995).

2. Consumerism
It has been suggested that a major challenge to the autonomy of health professionals derives from consumers of health care, who

are increasingly able to challenge the professional's expertise. Such challenges may arise from the fact that the public has greater access to, and better understanding of, medical knowledge, and that 'experts' are no longer revered and respected. This trend has been accelerated by the proliferation of information on medical issues both in the media and on the Internet. Such challenges to medical authority are especially evident in relation to the prescribing practices of general practitioners who sometimes feel that they have to take patient demands into account (Weiss and Fitzpatrick, 1997). It is possible, however, that these developments could enhance the authority of pharmacists. Consumers have ready access to a wider range of medicines than they did a decade ago. This is in part due to the deregulation for sale of a number of medicines which formerly could only be prescribed, which has the effect of enhancing consumer choice. It may also be intensified by the advent of direct-to-consumer advertising which has been facilitated by the Internet (Lexchin, 1999). While deregulation may reduce the autonomy of medical practitioners, it could potentially increase the scope and responsibility of pharmacists to work with patients in the management of the individual's own health (Britten, 2001). As people have greater choice and control over which drugs and therapies they want to buy, the pharmacist, arguably has a pivotal role to monitor their purchases. The Royal Pharmaceutical Society has long asserted that there is an important difference between the purchase of medicines and drugs and other commodities. Hibbert *et al.* (2002), in a study which empirically examines these issues, cites a Pharmaceutical Society report published in the 1940s which noted:

'Drugs and medicines are not ordinary commercial articles for which the limit of the market may safely be the desire and capacity of the public to purchase them. Moreover, medicines are products of which the public are unable to judge the quality and suitability for their purpose' (Pharmaceutical Society's Report of the Committee of Inquiry 1941 (Part 2), cited in Hibbert *et al.*, 2002)

What Hibbert and his colleagues found, however, when they interviewed both pharmacists and consumers, was that in practice the interactions between pharmacists and consumers tend to be routinised and that there is relatively little considered discussion between the professional and the client. Although pharmacists, or more often than not other counter staff, ask consumers questions associated with their planned use of the medicines, the interaction becomes almost ritualised. They conclude that:

'Protocol questioning would seem to routinise the pharmacist's knowledge base, such that aspects of the questioning can be delegated to less qualified staff. It does not therefore automatically equate with increased

scope for interpretative responses to individual consumers or greater opportunities to practise the professional "art"' (Hibbert *et al.*, 2002).

3. *Corporatisation of pharmacy*

Increasingly, community pharmacists are employed in pharmacies owned by large corporate organisations, whether they are multiple pharmacy chains or supermarkets. The necessarily bureaucratic nature of these organisations has contributed to what has been termed the McDonaldisation of pharmacy (see Chapter 2). Inevitably, as these large organisations seek to maximise efficiency and profitability, procedures and operations become routinised and products and services standardised (Ritzer, 2000). It can be argued that reducing opportunities for pharmacists to exercise independent professional judgement, as they become 'governed' by protocols and 'company policy', risks compromising their professional autonomy.

4. *Increasing dependence on technology*

In recent years, developments in computer technology, and the technology within the pharmaceutical industry to prepare and package medicines, have revolutionised pharmacists' daily activities.

The manufacturing role of pharmacists within hospital and community practice has been all but eliminated by the availability of medicines, formulated and manufactured by the pharmaceutical industry. Moreover, pharmacists today are rarely even required to count tablets or capsules, as patient packs in which convenient numbers of doses are supplied by the manufacturer in packages, complete with information inserts for the patient, is the norm. Thus, the time taken to dispense individual medicines is less than in the past, whilst concurrently the number of prescriptions dispensed per pharmacy increases steadily each year. Consequently, most of the 'mystique' the public has traditionally associated with the compounding aspects of the pharmacist's role, perhaps exemplified by the iconic status of the pestle and mortar, has largely disappeared. Nowadays, in both community and hospital pharmacy practice, the 'practical' aspects of dispensing are viewed as technical activities and are largely carried out by pharmacy technicians rather than by pharmacists. Indeed, several hospital pharmacies have gone one step further and introduced robotic dispensing systems, such that all mystique is removed from the dispensing process and pharmacists can be argued to have lost control over what has previously been considered their key activity. As we have illustrated above, the criteria for professional status depends on the profession maintaining a 'social distance' from the public it serves, and nowadays the pharmacist who remains in the dispensary may seem to the public to be no more than a supplier of pre-packaged medicines.

5. *Dependence on physicians and constraints on the pharmacist's authority*

To a great extent pharmacists receive their directions from physicians. It is they who make the assessment of a case from a clinical and therapeutic viewpoint, whilst pharmacists dispense in accordance with prescribers' wishes. Both in the hospital and particularly in the community environment, the pharmacist is 'governed' by the decisions and judgements of the medical profession. In day-to-day practice pharmacists are often reluctant to, or perhaps more accurately are discouraged from questioning the prescribing decisions of doctors (Harding *et al.*, 1994). More recently Edmunds and Calnan (2001) have suggested that this ceding of ultimate authority to doctors may hinder community pharmacists from achieving professional status. Pharmacists, while frequently characterised as medicines experts, have thus historically failed to exercise control over the medicines themselves. Denzin and Mettlin (1968) have claimed this *'failure to gain control over the social object which justifies existence of its professional qualities in the first place'* results in pharmacy being a case of incomplete professionalisation.

The increased use of pre-packaged medicines, computer technology and the dependence of pharmacists on the prescribers' judgement can be argued to have contributed to a shift in the pharmaceutical profession's I/T ratio, in that there is limited scope for pharmacists to bring their own unique knowledge and skills to their day-to-day tasks; that is to say, they are too highly trained for the jobs they do. Furthermore, Turner (1995) has argued that the specialised knowledge base of pharmacists is very precise and formulaic, lacking mystique. This contrasts sharply with the 'clinical mentality' which doctors constantly rely on when making decisions in the face of uncertainty.

Inter-professional working

The professional relationship between community pharmacists and other members of the primary health care team has long been distinct from that of other health care workers, largely because community pharmacies are commercial businesses as well as service providers. This, as we have seen, has led to considerable debate as to the precise professional status of community pharmacists in particular. Notwithstanding this function as business entrepreneurs, most community pharmacists have long-established relationships with other health care professions such as general practitioners and nurses. The characteristics of these relationships centre on pharmacists' specialist knowledge of drugs. Research into the relationships of pharmacists and GPs working together in health centres indicates that the pharmacists' role is considered complementary to those of other members of the primary health care team (Harding *et al.*, 1994). However, historically the integration of pharmacies into health centres has not been common, and GP surgeries and community pharmacies have largely evolved separate from one another. Recently, several developments in primary health care policy have introduced opportunities for pharmacists to more fully integrate their role into the primary health care team. The establishment of Primary Care Groups (PCGs), and latterly Primary Care Trusts (PCTs) in England, and their equivalents in Wales and Scotland, has created greater opportunities for pharmacists to work with GP practices as primary care pharmacists. GP drug expenditure represents approximately 50 per cent of the costs of primary care and pharmacists are increasingly seen as the team member with the appropriate expertise to help in the management and control of prescribing budgets (Mason, 1999). Another significant development is the proposed introduction of 500 'one stop primary health care centres' by 2004 (Department of Health, 2000). These centres will provide opportunities to integrate pharmacy services fully into primary care.

A further important recent development to impact on pharmacy has been the establishment of Personal Medical Services (PMS). Prior to its introduction, GPs were contracted by local health authorities to provide health care. As the contractors, GPs employed nurses, receptionists, etc. Under PMS health professionals other than GPs could bid to provide health care if they ensured that medical services were delivered by a general medical practitioner. This new arrangement has meant that in some instances, nurses have replaced GPs as the contract holders, with the nurses employing GPs. The possibility exists for pharmacists, too, to become contractors. Moreover, PMS shifts the emphasis of primary care away from a diagnostic/curative model, based on a hierarchy headed by the GP, and more towards a social health model with its emphasis on health maintenance adopted by the primary health care team as a whole. This shift fits with the remit of pharmacists to promote health. An example of this, drawn from an evaluation study of PMS, illustrates the impact of modifying traditional professional roles between pharmacists and GPs. In one PMS practice, the development of trust led to one GP sanctioning the local community pharmacist's autonomy to supervise methadone dispensing (Riley *et al.*, 2003).

The implications of these changing relationships are also evidenced by the introduction of policies to enable practitioners, other than GPs and dentists, to prescribe medicines. Specially trained pharmacists and nurses are to be allowed to become designated supplementary prescribers, prescribing, in the first instance, medication for asthmatics, diabetics, those with coronary heart disease and high blood pressure.

Notwithstanding these developments in primary care,

community pharmacists, in developing their role, will necessarily have to renegotiate areas of professional responsibility and confront the issue of 'boundary encroachment' whereby pharmacists may seek to assume roles traditionally performed by other health professionals, as with the case of pharmacist prescribing. Research evidence suggests that pharmacists view the development and extension of their professional role as a bid for survival rather than an attempt to usurp the role of general practitioners. However, many GPs, whilst accommodating some changes in community pharmacy, perceive some of the new initiatives as a threat to their autonomy and control (Edmunds and Calnan, 2001).

Pharmacy's status in the future

Professionalism is not an acquired state; rather it is a dynamic social process in a continual state of flux. For instance, following recent high-profile cases, the government has questioned the ability of all health professionals to self-regulate effectively. Consequently, more transparent and accountable regulatory frameworks and complaints procedures have been, or are being, introduced. Currently there are some important questions to be asked about the nature of pharmacists' activities and their contribution to the provision of health care. This will have implications for their relationships with other health professionals as well as for their relationships with consumers of health care and the State. One strategic response to challenges to their privileged status may be for professions to pursue what has been called a 'professional project' (Macdonald, 1995) to persuade the State and public of the

Table 7.1 Potential professional projects (adapted from Harding and Taylor, 2001)

Strategy	Advantages	Disadvantages
Improve consumers' access to pharmacist	Showcase for indeterminate knowledge	Devalues 'experts' time, diminishes mystique
Delegate dispensing duties to technicians	Reduced involvement in technical activities	Distances pharmacists from their traditional function
Increase advisory function	Increased opportunities to exercise professional judgement	May eclipse 'core dispensing functions'
Deliver pharmaceutical care (medicines management)	Defines boundaries of pharmacist's responsibility	Possible boundary encroachment with allied professionals, e.g. medical practitioners
Pharmacist prescribing	Use of clinical skills and judgement	Boundary encroachment, a completely 'new' role
Evidence-based service delivery	Delivers best practice	Constrains individual professional autonomy
Promote the symbolic value pharmacists add to medicines	Exclusive function of pharmacists	Ethereal and unevaluated

value of its work. In the case of pharmacy, it has been suggested that a professional project for pharmacy might include the strategies outlined in Table 7.1. These will afford opportunities for pharmacists to consolidate their privileged position by creating dependence, by the State and the public, on the services they offer. By developing such activities, including many which have been outlined in the so-called 'extended role' as detailed in Chapter 2, the opportunities exist for pharmacists to shed the image of over-educated, under-utilised health workers. This would in turn have the effect of increasing pharmacists' I/T ratio – that is, as pharmacists become increasingly involved in providing medicines management, health care advice and education, there will be a commensurate rise in their level of indeterminate knowledge. Moreover, a social distance would be created as the knowledge base and expertise of pharmacists demanded by the public and legitimised by the State is preserved and protected.

SUMMARY

- Professions possess certain key characteristics or traits
- Professionals fulfil important societal functions
- Pharmacy exhibits the characteristics of a profession as outlined by the 'trait theory'
- Many factors hinder pharmacists' professional autonomy
- Pharmacists increasingly work in an integrated way with other health care professionals
- Professionalism is a dynamic social and political process.

FURTHER READING

Anderson, S. (2001) The historical context of pharmacy. In: K.M.G. Taylor and G. Harding (eds) *Pharmacy Practice*, London, Taylor and Francis, pp. 3–30.

Edmunds, J. and Calnan, M.W. (2001) The reprofessionalisation of community pharmacy? An exploration of attitudes to extended roles for community pharmacists amongst pharmacists and general practitioners in the United Kingdom. *Social Science and Medicine*, 53, 943–955.

Holloway, S.W.F. (1991) *Royal Pharmaceutical Society of Great Britain 1841–1991. A Political and Social History*, London, The Pharmaceutical Press.

Macdonald, K.M. (1995) *The Sociology of the Professions*, London, Sage Publications.

Turner, B.S. (1995) *Medical Power and Social Knowledge* (2nd edn), London, Sage Publications.

REFERENCES

Britten, N. (2001) Prescribing and the defence of clinical autonomy. *Sociology of Health and Illness*, 23, 478–496.

Denzin, N.K. and Mettlin, C.J. (1968) Incomplete professionalisation: the case of pharmacy. *Social Forces*, 46, 375–381.

Department of Health (2000) *The NHS Plan: A Plan for Investment. A Plan for Reform*. London, Stationery Office.

Dingwall, R. and Wilson, E. (1995) Is pharmacy really an incomplete profession? *Perspectives on Social Problems*, 7, 111–128.

Edmunds, J. and Calnan, M.W. (2001) The reprofessionalisation of community pharmacy? An exploration of attitudes to extended roles for community pharmacists amongst pharmacists and general practitioners in the United Kingdom. *Social Science and Medicine*, 53, 943–955.

Freidson, E. (1970a) *Profession of Medicine: A Study in the Sociology of Applied Knowledge*, New York, Dodd Mead.

Freidson, E. (1970b) *Professional Dominance*, Chicago, Atherton Press.

Goode, W.J. (1960) Encroachment, charlatanism and the emerging profession: psychiatry, sociology and medicine. *American Sociological Review*, 25, 902–914.

Harding, G. and Taylor, K.M.G (2001) Pharmacy as a profession. In: K.M.G. Taylor and G. Harding (eds) *Pharmacy Practice*, London, Taylor and Francis, pp. 187–202.

Harding, G., Taylor, K.M.G. and Nettleton, S. (1994) Working for health: interprofessional relations in health centres. In: G. Harding, S. Nettleton and K.M.G. Taylor (eds) *Social Pharmacy: Innovation and Change*, London, Pharmaceutical Press.

Hibbert, D., Bissell, P. and Ward, P.R. (2002) Consumerism and professional work in the community pharmacy. *Sociology of Health and Illness*, 24, 46–65.

Jamous, H. and Peloille, B. (1970) Changes in the French university hospital system. In: J.A. Jackson (ed.) *Professions and Professionalisation*, Cambridge, Cambridge University Press, pp. 110–152.

Johnson, T. (1989) *Professions and Power*, London, Macmillan Education Ltd.

King, M.D. (1968) Science and the professional dilemma. In: J. Gould (ed) *Penguin Social Sciences Survey*, Harmondsworth, Penguin.

Lexchin, J. (1999) Direct-to-consumer advertising: impact upon patient expectations regarding disease management. *Disease Management and Health Outcomes*, 5, 273–283.

Macdonald, K.M. (1995) *The Sociology of the Professions*, London, Sage Publications.

Mason, P. (1999) Opportunities for pharmacists in primary care. *Primary Care Pharmacy*, 1, 3–5.

Parsons, T. (1939) The professions and the social structure. *Social Forces*, 17, 457–467.

Riley, A.J., Harding, G., Meads, G., Underwood, M. and Carter, Y.H. (2003) The times they are a changin': An evaluation of Personal Medical Services Pilots. *Journal of Inter-professional Care*, 17, 127–139.

Ritzer, G. (2000) *The McDonaldization of Society* (2nd edn), Thousand Oaks, Calif., Pine Forge Press.

Shuval, J.T. (1981) The contribution of psychology and social phenomena to an understanding of the aetiology of disease and illness. *Social Science and Medicine*, 15, 337–342.

Turner, B.S. (1995) *Medical Power and Social Knowledge* (2nd edn), London, Sage Publications.

Weiss, M. and Fitzpatrick, R. (1997) Challenges to medicine: the case of prescribing. *Sociology of Health and Illness*, 19, 297–327.

Wright, P. (1979) A study of the legitimisation of knowledge: the success of medicine and the failure of astrology. In: R. Wallis (ed.) *On the Margins of Science*, Sociological Review Monograph 27, Keele, University of Keele, pp. 85–101.

Maintaining and Promoting Health

INTRODUCTION

Health promotion and disease prevention together comprise one of the key elements of Good Pharmacy Practice as outlined by the World Health Organisation and the International Pharmaceutical Federation (FIP) (Box 8.1).

Box 8.1 Elements of Good Pharmacy Practice (WHO, 1996)

- Health promotion and disease prevention
- Supply and use of medicines
- Self-care
- Influencing prescribing

Educating people about the prevention of ill-health and encouraging them to act upon this information is a complex process. A sociological perspective can help pharmacists understand how people relate to health, illness and disease. It can also contribute to an understanding of the political context in which policies on the promotion of health and the prevention of disease are developed and implemented. In this chapter we will examine a number of approaches to health promotion and consider some of the obstacles health professionals face in attempting to promote healthy lifestyles. Effective health promotion also requires a behavioural and psychological understanding of human behaviour. Whilst these aspects are necessarily touched upon in this chapter, for a greater understanding of a behavioural approach to health promotion in a pharmacy setting, readers are referred to McClelland and Rees (2000). Moreover, it is not our intention here to highlight all the opportunities available for health promotion within pharmacies. For detail of the development and delivery of pharmacy-based health promotion schemes, readers should refer to Blenkinsopp *et al.* (2000).

The community pharmacist is frequently highlighted as being well placed to offer opportunistic health education and health promotion to the public. Since the early 1960s, community pharmacies have been recognised as being ideally located within the community for the provision of health education. The Nuffield Report (Nuffield Committee of Inquiry into Pharmacy, 1986), Pharmacy in a New Age (Royal Pharmaceutical Society of Great Britain, 1996, 1997) and recent government policy (Department of Health, 2000), have all envisaged a development of pharmacists' activities in the community, with pharmacists becoming more actively involved in advising patients about prescribed and purchased medication and providing advice and education on general health matters.

Since the early 1980s, illness prevention, rather than cure, has become a major priority in health policy. This has been the result of a combination of factors, including a growing appreciation of the limitations of conventional medical practice (see Chapter 5), an increasing concern about the rapidly increasing costs of health care services associated with the insatiable demand for health care, and the changing nature of the disease burden. Today, in countries which have passed through the so-called 'epidemiological transition', people are more likely to die from chronic conditions, which are largely preventable, than they are from infectious diseases. Heart disease, cancers and accidents are some of the major killers in our society and can, to a great extent, be prevented. The World Health Organisation is also committed to prevention and the UK, along with other European countries, has agreed to develop policies which are in line with the strategies outlined in its document *Health 21: The Health for all Policy Framework for the WHO European Region* (WHO, 1998).

The two main stated aims in the document are:

1. To promote and protect people's health throughout their lives.
2. To reduce the incidence of the main diseases and injuries, and alleviate the suffering they cause.

Implicit in the strategies of health promotion which encourage people to take responsibility for the maintenance and preservation of their own health, is the hope that there will be a subsequent reduction in demand for health services. Successive governments have been eager to adopt a preventive approach to health care. This has been outlined in a series of government documents detailing the merits of preventive health strategies and health promotion. Two major themes run through these reports. First, a recognised need to reduce the demands on public spending; second, an emphasis on the contribution individuals can make to improve their own health status.

The White Paper *Promoting Better Health* (Department of Health, 1987) emphasised the importance of health promotion in primary health care, and indicated that in future community pharmacists would be remunerated for services other than dispensing prescriptions. The *Health of the Nation* (Department of Health, 1992) highlighted the importance of health promotion and multi-disciplinary collaboration in the reduction of morbidity and mortality from coronary heart disease, cancer, mental illness/suicide, HIV/AIDS and sexual health, and accidents. Targets were set in each of these areas, to be achieved through lifestyle changes in the areas of smoking, diet and nutrition, blood pressure and HIV/AIDS associated with injecting drug misuse. *Primary Care:*

The Future (Department of Health, 1996) called for the development, nationally, of health promotion delivered from pharmacies, and emphasised that pharmacists should be promoting health in order for *Health of the Nation* targets to be met.

Whilst preventive measures are generally considered to be desirable, the approach to prevention and health was the focus of much debate. The policies outlined above focused on the lifestyles of individuals. The strategy caused a great deal of controversy and was challenged by those who argued that it failed to address the real determinants of health, which are seen to lie in social and economic factors. Poverty, poor housing and food policies, for example, would seem to be more important considerations in promoting health than 'healthy eating' or taking 'regular exercise'. The circumstances which permit or enable people to live healthy lives are an essential prerequisite to healthy lifestyles. In other words, the divergent approaches to preventive health policy are closely allied to our interpretation or explanation of the relationship between social factors and health (Chapter 6). For instance, to assume that everyone can adopt a healthy lifestyle, i.e. partake of a balanced diet, sufficient exercise and so forth, fails to take into account the individual's immediate circumstances and the environment in which they live, which may actually prevent the adoption of such lifestyles.

A change in political complexion with the New Labour landslide election victory in 1997 resulted in a different approach to health promotion and public health policies. Whilst previous governments had emphasised the importance of individual behaviours and personal responsibility for health, New Labour espoused a different approach, which they call the 'Third Way'. In the context of health promotion and illness prevention, the third way comprises a 'contract' between individuals, local communities/organisations and national government. Perhaps the most important change was that the issue of health inequalities was placed near the top of the health policy agenda. As we saw in Chapter 6, the Minister of Public Health set up an independent commission to investigate the matter (Acheson Report, 1998), and the government pledged to reduce health inequalities and fight poverty and social exclusion. To this end, a series of policy initiatives were introduced and implemented. These include fiscal policies to reduce poverty amongst households with children (e.g. the working families and child care tax credits), the National Strategy for Neighbourhood Renewal, the multi-agency Sure Start Programme designed to bring education, health and social services together to improve the lives of children living in disadvantaged areas, and other area initiatives such as Health Action Zones.

Policy documents such as *The New NHS: Modern, Dependable* (Department of Health, 1997) and *Our Healthier Nation* (Department of Health, 1998) also focus on how health care providers, including pharmacists, can contribute to the population's health, whilst being particularly concerned with reducing the health-gap between rich and poor. The government has attempted to shift the balance of power from acute services to primary care. For example, Primary Care Trusts have a key role to play in the development and implementation of public health policies – by way of community development work, health promotion, health education and commissioning for services for better health.

Pharmacists, as players in the new public health movement, are now expected to provide support and advice for people to help them take responsibility for maintaining their own health, for instance by offering dietary advice, cholesterol testing, and helping to minimise the health risks associated with injecting illicit substances. To be a pharmacist is to be an effective health promoter. However, this requires pharmacists to appreciate that part of the 'arrangement' whereby people accept responsibility and some control over their own health is that these people are also empowered to question health professionals. An empowered population responsible for its own health maintenance is also empowered to question and reject health professional advice and information. As Martin and McQueen (1989) have observed the *essence of the new public health is a healthy scepticism about the role that health professionals, whether biomedical or behaviourally based, can play in the reduction and amelioration of ill health . . .'*

Alongside a prioritisation of health inequalities, developing partnerships and multi-agency working and shifting the balance of power to primary care, the contemporary policy agenda is dominated by the need to provide evidence for the effectiveness of interventions. The Health Development Agency (formally the Health Education Authority) and the NHS Centre for Reviews and Dissemination are two examples of organisations which have been charged with the remit of evaluating the effectiveness of health interventions and health promotion initiatives. Evidence-based medicine and health care is important because we need to know whether or not health promotion and health education activities actually work (see Chapter 5).

PREVENTING ILL-HEALTH

It will be useful at this point to outline what we mean by prevention in relation to ill-health. In health policy, it is generally accepted that there are three levels or dimensions to prevention.

1. *Primary prevention*: action to prevent the occurrence of disease or disability – for example, immunisation and vaccination, improved sanitation, water fluoridisation, better housing and

nutrition. Within the NHS, services mainly concerned with primary prevention include family planning, immunisation schemes, health education and health visiting. Examples of health prevention outside the NHS would include clean air and seat belt legislation, environmental health, the Health and Safety at Work Act, and the factory inspectorate.

2. *Secondary prevention*: the early detection of a condition which if detected may be treated. This form of preventive activity may include dental examinations, eye testing, periodic medical examinations, and screening techniques – for example, blood pressure measuring, blood glucose and cholesterol testing, and cervical smears.

3. *Tertiary prevention*: minimising disability arising out of existing conditions. This may involve care or rehabilitation for conditions such as hearing impairment, diabetes, epilepsy, mental disorder and spinal injuries.

The increasing emphasis on prevention has significant implications for the health professions. The government has repeatedly pointed to the contribution that health professionals, particularly those in primary care, can make to health prevention and health promotion. Indeed, since the Nuffield Inquiry into Pharmacy, health promoting and advising activities have become a cornerstone of strategies for pharmacists' professional development.

Let us consider what is understood by the terms 'health education' and 'health promotion', and reflect briefly on the philosophy underlying health education.

HEALTH EDUCATION

It is possible to identify three aspects of health education (Box 8.2).

• Education about the human body and how to look after it
• Education about health services and information about the availability of services and their use
• Consideration of the wider environment, where information can be disseminated, and changes effected with respect to matters such as pollution and clean water

Box 8.2 Aspects of health education

Health education has been defined in many ways. The definition offered by Catford and Nutbeam (1984) is instructive:

'[Health education] seeks to improve or protect health through voluntary changes in behaviour as a consequence of learning opportunities. It can include personal education and development, and mass media information and education.'

In other words, the aim of health educators is to encourage people to change their behaviour and adopt health activities with a view to improving their health status. Education can take place at personal, community, and societal levels.

Tones (1986) identified three approaches to health education. All are still practised to a greater or lesser extent, although the order in which they are presented here reflects the historical development of approaches to health education.

1. *Traditional health education*

The traditional health education approach is based on the belief that the incidence of ill-health can be reduced considerably if individuals adopt a healthy lifestyle. Health education has therefore traditionally been designed to persuade individuals to replace their unhealthy patterns of behaviour with mostly healthy ones. Hence the task of health educators has been, for example, to persuade people to drink less alcohol, stop smoking, and reduce their consumption of saturated fats, on the grounds that doing so would promote their health. This approach has obvious financial attractions for health educators in so far as the savings accruing from a reduction in demand for health care services would far outweigh the cost of a persuasive health education campaign.

2. *Educational model*

The educational model of health education is less didactic in approach. Its underlying principle is that individuals should be educated, not about specific health issues but about decision-making skills, in order that they can make informed choices about their health-related behaviour. However, as Tones argues, this model is not without its criticisms. The impact of socialisation may mean that a rational decision competes with cultural influences in making decisions. For instance, individuals addicted to drugs may be fully aware of the risks to their health from drug misuse, but may not be in a position to stop their drug taking because of the social milieu in which they live. Similarly, an adolescent's decision to smoke may be made by reference to cultural or peer decision-making processes which 'rationalise' smoking as 'tough', 'glamorous' or even 'a stimulant' to help cope with living in a dreary environment. Failure to make the rational choice – to give up smoking for health reasons – can lead to a situation of 'victim blaming' by health educators, as individuals are blamed for failing to make the 'required' health-promoting decisions.

3. *Radical model*

As we have already discussed in Chapter 6, ill-health is not simply a matter of chance, but rather is related to social factors. However, an assumption of the 'radical model' is that through changing people's social circumstances individuals can be empowered to take control over the factors that influence their health. This may be achieved, first, by raising their awareness of the obstacles to health and, second, by individuals taking positive action against these obstacles. For example, air pollution from heavy industrial processing plants situated next to a residential area may be a significant contributor to a high local incidence of chest diseases. The 'radical' model advocates people to become aware of the adverse effects of such an industry on their health, and encourages concerned individuals to take collective action against the cause of ill-health. In essence, then, this model is 'radical' in that it attempts to make health education a political issue by encouraging people to use their collective power to promote health.

The limitations of the 'traditional' or 'educational' approach to health education were clearly articulated by Rodmell and Watt (1986) in their book *The Politics of Health Education*. They have challenged the traditional health education approach on five counts.

1. Traditional health education 'individualises' health, i.e. the preservation of health is considered by health educators as the responsibility of the individual.
2. 'Elitism'. An implicit assumption of the traditional health education philosophy is an absence or inappropriateness of the lay person's own health knowledge, thus health educators may assume that their interpretation of health and illness is better or more appropriate than the interpretation of lay people. Consequently, health education programmes can be insensitive to socio-cultural variations in health knowledge, or ride rough-shod over them.
3. Health education is frequently imposed on individuals without the message being tailored to their needs, i.e. they may not be told what they want or need to know, but rather what the education programme wants to teach. Therefore, the health education package is separated from the needs of the individual. However, failure to pick up on this inappropriate health education message is often deemed to be the result of the recipient's irresponsibility or intransigence.
4. The dominant value system in society is used as a vehicle to promote health. That is, health education, like media advertising, relies on the use of images. These images, however, are frequently reflections of affluent, white, middle-class lifestyles. The values implicit in these images may be totally unrelated or divorced from the lifestyles of the targeted audience.
5. The agenda for health education is not always determined strictly in accordance with health needs. It is drawn up on the basis of political decisions about the allocation of scarce financial resources, and this agenda may be drafted by individuals

whose life experiences may be far removed from, and have little in common with, the targeted population.

Throughout the 1980s the more radical approach to health education, discussed above, came to be referred to as health promotion.

HEALTH PROMOTION

The term 'health promotion' is used to mean different things by different people, including health professionals. In practice, many people often equate health promotion with health education. However, it is desirable to maintain a distinction between the two terms, to ensure that the non-educational elements of health promotion are not overlooked (Downie *et al.*, 1996).

Health promotion involves the various means which enable or facilitate people to preserve and/or maintain their health. Catford and Nutbeam (1984) define health promotion as that which:

'seeks to improve or protect health through behavioural, biological, socio-economical and environmental changes. It can include health education, personal services, environmental measures, community and organisational development and economic regulatory activities.'

Thus health promotion is more than simply dissemination of information and would involve attempts to influence the activities, for example, of employers and local authorities. Tannahill (1985) has developed a model of health promotion which encompasses three overlapping spheres of activity: health education, prevention and health protection. This model, shown in Figure 8.1, is intended to be illustrative rather than rigid, and reveals seven domains distinguishable within health promotion. Such a model provides a starting point for the defining, planning and delivery of health promotion.

Summarising this model, Downie *et al.* (1996) have proposed an alternative definition:

'Health promotion comprises efforts to enhance positive health and reduce the risk of ill-health, through the overlapping spheres of health education, prevention and health protection.'

It is important that pharmacists, who are being encouraged to participate more actively in health promotion, are aware of what is involved at both a practical and philosophical level. Simply telling health professionals to become health promoters can be counter-productive for both the consumers and providers of health care. For instance, supplying sterile injecting equipment to drug misusers from community pharmacies has been promoted as

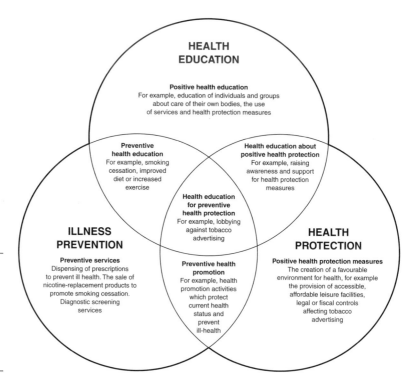

Figure 8.1
Tannahill's model of health promotion (reproduced with permission from McClelland and Rees, 2000)

The figure contains the following labelled areas:

HEALTH EDUCATION

Positive health education
For example, education of individuals and groups about care of their own bodies, the use of services and health protection measures

Preventive health education
For example, smoking cessation, improved diet or increased exercise

Health education about positive health protection
For example, raising awareness and support for health protection measures

Health education for preventive health protection
For example, lobbying against tobacco advertising

ILLNESS PREVENTION

Preventive services
Dispensing of prescriptions to prevent ill health. The sale of nicotine-replacement products to promote smoking cessation. Diagnostic screening services

Preventive health promotion
For example, health promotion activities which protect current health status and prevent ill-health

HEALTH PROTECTION

Positive health protection measures
The creation of a favourable environment for health, for example the provision of accessible, affordable leisure facilities, legal or fiscal controls affecting tobacco advertising

an appropriate harm minimisation strategy for this client group. Nevertheless, many pharmacists are resistant to taking on such an activity, viewing it as problematic (for instance, resulting in thefts from their pharmacy) and likely to be perceived negatively by their 'regular' clients (Rees *et al.*, 1997).

Sociologically informed literature on health promotion and pharmacy is relatively limited. Health promotion has in the past often been conceived primarily in terms of advice-giving in response to the presentation of symptoms. However, with the advent of pharmacy-based health promotion schemes, providing advice and information on (for instance) drug misuse, dental health, diet, and smoking cessation, and their subsequent evaluation, some data is becoming available. McClelland and Rees (2000) have classified pharmacists' health-promoting activities into primary, secondary and tertiary activities in a manner consistent with the definitions of primary, secondary and tertiary prevention, outlined opposite (see Table 8.1).

More has been written on opportunistic health education and health promotion in relation to medical general practice. A particularly instructive paper is Watt's (1986) 'Community Health Initiatives and their relationship to general practice'. Watt points to the development and proliferation of community health initiatives, which fall into three categories:

Target area	Primary health promotion	Secondary health promotion	Tertiary health promotion
Coronary heart disease and strokes	Smoking cessation Weight reduction	Blood pressure monitoring Cholesterol testing	Adherence to medication Adoption and maintenance of healthy lifestyle
HIV/AIDS and sexual health	Contraception Safe sexual practices	HIV screening	Adherence to medication
Cancer	Sunscreens Smoking cessation	Cervical screening Mammography	Prosthesis service Self–help and support group
Accidents	Supply of childproof devices		Aids for those with physical disability
Mental health	Increased awareness of predisposing factors		Adherence to medication Decreased stigma
Environment	Improve working environment		

Table 8.1 Possible targets for pharmacists in primary, secondary and tertiary health promotion (reproduced with permission from McClelland and Rees, 2000)

1. Self-help groups, where *'people who either suffer from a condition or are relatives of a sufferer, meet together to give each other mutual support'*.
2. Community help groups are locally based groups which recognise and address the importance of social factors to health. Watt gives the following example: *'Women on a housing estate who share a state of depression, and who identify its cause as isolation which in turn is caused by there being nowhere safe for small children to play, decide to treat the depression by campaigning for play space.'*
3. Community development health projects are usually local authority funded projects that are focused on a specific health issue. The principal aim is to encourage and facilitate participation in that people should have a far greater say in the conditions in which they live. *'While community development health projects vary widely, one common element is the understanding that health is not an individual matter. Participants in community development health projects identify the causes of ill health in certain social factors over which individuals have little control.'*

Watt suggests there is scope for useful links to be formed between these initiatives and general practitioners, and she offers suggestions as to how general practitioners may contribute to community health schemes. These suggestions are worthy of consideration by pharmacists who are community based and may well be in a position to contribute to such health promotion initiatives. Scope for the involvement of pharmacists in health promotion and public health has been enhanced by the emphasis that has been placed on the public health function of Primary Care Trusts, and in particular in their efforts to implement their Health Improvement Programmes. Suggestions which may be of particular relevance for community pharmacists include:

1. Taking into consideration patients' own experiences, interpretations, and perceived health needs may enable health practitioners to offer more effective support.
2. Health practitioners should be aware of and become involved in, 'local informal health networks'. For example, the Community Health Council, the Council for Voluntary Service, and local self-help groups.
3. Health practitioners might serve as a resource for community based groups, for example offering to give informal talks to such groups.

Approaches to health promotion

There are many ways of defining health promotion, and a multiplicity of approaches. These have been usefully summarised by Beattie (1991) in the typology, illustrated in Figure 8.2.

Beattie's schema is based on two dichotomies: first, the 'mode of intervention' which may be either authoritative or negotiated; second, the 'focus of intervention' which may be aimed at influencing individuals or groups of people. On the basis of these dimensions he then identifies four approaches to health promotion:

1. 'Health persuasion techniques' – these are interventions which employ the authority of public health expertise to redirect the behaviour of individuals in top-down prescriptive ways. This strategy has a long history, and traditional forms of health

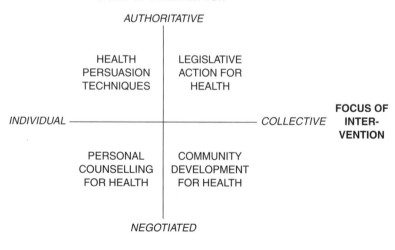

Figure 8.2 Beattie's strategies for health promotion (Beattie, 1991)

education would fall into this category – for example, the sexually transmitted disease campaigns deployed during the First World War and the mass media AIDS campaigns of the early 1980s. 'Ask your Pharmacist' campaigns, where the public is exhorted to consult community pharmacists, are another such example. Governments may favour this approach because of its high profile and it can be relatively inexpensive. However, there is evidence that it is not necessarily cost-effective.

2. 'Legislative action for health' is where the authority of public health expertise is drawn upon to influence legislation. Examples of this approach would include Clean Air Acts, compulsory fluoridation of water supplies, control over tobacco advertising and restrictions on the pack size of analgesics containing paracetamol that may be purchased over the counter.

3. A negotiated approach which is oriented towards individuals is 'personal counselling for health'. This approach involves the use of individual or group counselling to encourage people to reflect upon and thereby be encouraged to alter their lifestyles. It has become more common in general medical practice, and indeed private counselling areas are becoming increasingly incorporated into community pharmacies.

4. 'Community development for health' involves group-based action which aims to challenge conventional forms of health care and identify alternative means to promote health. This approach forms the basis of many of the neighbourhood renewal projects such as Sure Start which aims to bring various agencies and services together to work alongside and to foster local communities. On a smaller scale, food co-operatives provide an illustration of this approach. Food co-ops bring together volunteers and a number of outlets who are able to work together to pool their purchasing power and can then buy directly from wholesalers or farmers. For example, the Sandwell food co-op in the West Midlands brings together thirty-one outlets which supply fresh fruit and vegetables at a relatively cheap price to local residents (Petts, 2002).

Sociological analyses of health promotion

The identification of the various approaches to health promotion mapped out above using Beattie's typology represents a sociological analysis of the policy and organisational developments in health promotion. It is helpful in that it enables us to assess the merits and demerits of various strategies and their potential value for different health issues. The typology encompasses two divergent perspectives on health promotion. These perspectives reflect the two models of health and illness outlined in Chapter 5. At the risk of oversimplification, one perspective assumes that the individual can be held totally responsible for their own behaviour, while the other recognises that there are social constraints on the individual's actions. Such constraints have been reported in a study of health care routines in the family by Graham (1984), who makes a distinction between health choices and health compromises. The notion of choice is one that is central to health education. The theory is that people, when given information and advice (for example on diet, smoking or exercise), are placed in a position to choose whether or not to follow that advice. In practice, however, Graham's research revealed that the idea of being able to choose was often unrealistic and that in fact responding to such advice meant having to make compromises; that is, individuals weigh up the costs and benefits of responding to a health education message.

Bewley *et al.* (1984) in a study of adolescents' attitudes to illness and health, identified a number of social and health care problems experienced by young people living in an inner city area. Family disharmony compounded by poor housing and a lack of educational and employment opportunities was frequently reported by young people as among some of the problems they faced, and 'getting away' was considered the best solution. This situation, Bewley noted, illustrates the inappropriateness of the didactic approach of traditional health education which fails to take into account the target audience's socio-economic environment. Many of Bewley's respondents were aware of the chances they were taking with their health, but they were not prepared to do anything about some risks such as smoking. From their own perspective, preventive health behaviour was relegated low down their list of priorities, whilst they continued to live in an environment where coping with the daily problems of inner-city life were given uppermost priority.

The limitations that this imposes on the scope of traditional forms of health education are formidable. A way of acknowledging these limitations is to take account of, and draw upon, people's previous health experiences. That is to say, the way a person defines their state of health is through drawing on past knowledge and experience of health and illness, as discussed in Chapter 3. For instance, in response to a patient requesting excessive quantities of laxatives, a pharmacist may recommend an increase in the intake of dietary fibre. This advice, although therapeutically sound, may be inadequate if it takes no account of the patient's personal and social circumstances – that is, who purchases the food in their household, how much money is available for food, time available for purchase and preparation of food, food preferences of self and family – nor of their existing health beliefs – for example, their traditionally held beliefs on the merits of laxatives. All these factors come into play in the process of health promotion.

So it can be seen, then, that there are two approaches to health promotion which differ in their emphasis. These are not mutually exclusive. It is important that pharmacists' policy and practice of health education fully appreciates that it is inadequate merely to provide information in a didactic manner on the assumption that all individuals will respond in the same way. Rather, a health promotion policy should reflect an awareness of the attitudes, values and circumstances of those people to whom the policy is aimed.

Making sense of health promotion campaigns

In the 1980s, a national health promotion campaign was orchestrated in Wales to try to reduce the numbers of deaths from heart disease. 'Heart Beat Wales' was a multi-agency programme that not only provided the public with information on healthy lifestyles but also worked with commercial, government and voluntary organisations to ensure that the circumstances were such that people were better able to live healthier lives. An anthropologist evaluated this campaign and identified a number of important findings in terms of how people responded to and made sense of these promotional activities.

The promotional campaign highlighted the risks associated with heart disease. It identified these as being: eating too much fat, being obese, smoking, drinking too much alcohol, having high blood pressure, having insufficient exercise, and so on. When the anthropologist and his colleagues (Davison et al., 1991) spent time talking to the residents in Wales they found that these risk factors were well known to them. However, what people also know is that some people who are at the greatest risk of heart disease – that is overweight, heavy drinkers and smokers who have a bad diet – often live to a ripe old age, while other people, who are healthy, slim, non-smokers and 'into' healthy foods die of heart attacks. Thus, very often our empirical observations contradict the health promotion advice. In fact, as Davison points out, we all have 'an Uncle Norman' in that most of us can think of a person who is a 'heart attack waiting to happen' and yet never appears to become ill. Davison et al. (1991) concluded therefore that people collectively develop a 'lay epidemiology' which recognises that not all candidates have heart attacks and some non-candidates do, and that this must therefore be a question of luck. Health promoters, keen to present unequivocal, simplified and straightforward messages, fail to address these anomalies and so underestimate the sophistication of lay thinking. Davison et al conclude that it 'is ironic that such evidently fatalistic cultural concepts should be given more rather than less explanatory power by the activities of modern health education, whose stated goals lie in the opposite direction' (Davison et al., 1991).

PHARMACY AND HEALTH PROMOTION

The National Pharmaceutical Association's 'Ask your pharmacist, you'll be taking good advice' campaign, launched in 1983, was the first nationwide attempt to promote pharmacists as providers of health education advice. Television, magazine, leaflet and poster advertisements were employed to encourage people to consult the pharmacist on matters of health education and in particular to seek advice on the treatment of certain symptoms and minor illnesses. From 1986 the Department of Health funded the distribution of health care material by pharmacies through the 'Health Care in the High Street' (1986) and the 'Pharmacy Health Care' (1989) schemes. These schemes were joint initiatives of the Royal Pharmaceutical Society of Great Britain, Health Education Authority, Scottish Health Education Group, National Pharmaceutical Association and Family Planning Association and have involved the provision of health education literature and display stands to all community pharmacies. Literature supplied through the 'Health care in the high street' scheme has covered a variety of areas, including family planning, coronary heart disease, drug abuse, cystitis and AIDS. Since 1992, the scheme has been run by a company as the Pharmacy Health Care Scheme. Since 1994, the NHS contract for pharmaceutical services has provided for community pharmacies to be remunerated for displaying health promotion literature.

It is estimated that over six million people visit pharmacists every day, so pharmacists are in an ideal position to provide information, advice and support to patients, consumers and other health professionals (Blenkinsopp et al., 2000). As we have already seen in Chapter 3, the majority of symptoms experienced by people remain untreated. Pharmacists, then, have an important role in assisting patients with the purchase and use of medicines by supplying appropriate advice and information, whether solicited or not, and by determining if the symptoms experienced by a patient are sufficiently serious to merit a visit to their general practitioner.

Researchers involved with the development and evaluation of health promotion have proposed two levels of activity for pharmacists (Anderson, 2000). Level one refers to pharmacists encouraging healthy behaviour through the provision of verbal and written information and advice on healthy lifestyles and treating symptoms. Level two refers to more enduring and ongoing support with individuals and groups to help them to develop their health potential. In practice level two health promotion is likely to be most effective where pharmacists work with other health professionals and focus on areas where there is evidence of effectiveness. Successful areas of health promotion interventions involving pharmacists include smoking cessation, lipid management in the prevention of coronary heart disease, immunisation and emergency contraception (Blenkinsopp *et al.*, 2000).

Studies of pharmacy-based health education campaigns are limited and have often been oriented towards the prevention of disease and illness rather than the promotion of health *per se*. Health education has thus been rather narrowly defined, focusing on advice on symptoms and enhancing patient compliance. For example, the report *The Pharmacist as a Health Educator* (Shafford and Sharpe, 1989) concentrated predominantly on the advice given by pharmacists relating to symptoms and prescribed and non-prescribed medicines. In responding to symptoms, pharmacists may diagnose and if necessary treat a minor illness by sale of an over-the-counter (OTC) medicine and, where appropriate, refer patients to a general practitioner.

FROM COMPLIANCE TO CONCORDANCE

In addition to dealing with patient queries regarding symptoms or the use of specific purchased or dispensed medication, pharmacists, at the point of handing over a dispensed medicine, may reiterate the prescribers' instructions and give additional information when appropriate. This reinforcement of the prescribers' instructions may enhance the adherence of patients with the prescribed drug regimen. This ability to improve patient adherence is often quoted as an important facet of the pharmacist's role. However, it should be appreciated that the reasons for non-adherence of a patient with their prescribed drug regimen are many and varied.

The term 'adherence' is usually employed to describe a patient's use of medication in accordance with the directions of the prescriber. A broader definition might be the extent to which the patient's behaviour appears to be in accord with medical advice; this definition would consider whether the patient's lifestyle is also modified in accordance with professional health care advice. Adherence tends now to be used in place of the traditional term 'compliance', which is associated with a more paternalistic model of patient–health professional relations, in which the prescriber decides what is best for a client and they, in turn, are expected to comply with that decision.

A failure to follow medical advice is termed 'non-adherence' (or non-compliance) and may be either the result of a conscious decision (for instance, deliberately not taking medication), or unintentional due to a lack of appropriate information or a misunderstanding of how to medicate correctly. Failure to comply may result in a number of outcomes, including a worsening, or lack of improvement in the patient's condition, possibly with a concurrent increase in suffering. Non-adherence may also result in the occurrence of adverse effects, drug interactions and overdoses, and will also result in unnecessary wastage of costly health care resources. When dispensing medication the pharmacist is the last health care professional the patient encounters before commencing medication, and thus they potentially have a major input into ensuring patient adherence.

Recently the term 'concordance' has been introduced as a response to the changed relationship between the public and health care providers to denote the need for agreement between an individual and health professional relating to their illness and treatment. No longer is it considered appropriate for doctors and pharmacists to tell the public how to take their medicines correctly, rather the public are actively invited to participate in the professional's decision-making regarding medicine-taking.

A review of the literature covering fourteen studies, with a total of more than 10,000 patients, found an average rate of adherence of 64 per cent with antihypertensive therapy, with a range of 38–95 per cent (Dunbar-Jacob, 1991). A number of factors have been suggested as contributing to high levels of non-adherence (Box 8.3). Some of these are related to the drug and the dosing regimen, including patient misunderstanding of the directions given by the prescriber or on a medicine label, no immediate relief of symptoms, complex drug regimens with a large number of drugs being taken, and the occurrence of adverse effects. For instance, it has been estimated that 90 per cent of patients using inhaled steroids for the long-term treatment of bronchial asthma fail to comply properly with their prescribed therapy (Pharmaceutical Journal, 1989).

There are many important factors influencing adherence not directly related to the drug regimen, such as socio-economic factors, patient health beliefs, illness behaviour and the quality of the health professional/patient relationship (Chapter 4). For instance, the belief that a medicine is effective in treating a disease is likely to result in the patient following the prescribed regimen,

Box 8.3 Possible causes of intentional and unintentional non-adherence (adapted from Blenkinsopp *et al.*, 2000)

Intentional
- Denial of the diagnosis
- Patient's risk-benefit analysis not in favour of medicine-taking
- Medicine-taking places restrictions on lifestyle
- Differences in beliefs between patient and health professional

Unintentional
- Lack of knowledge regarding condition and its treatment
- Impaired vision
- Poor manual dexterity
- Problems with dosage form, e.g. inability to swallow tablets, or poor inhaler technique
- Forgetfulness
- Adverse effects
- Confusion with complex medication regime

whilst scepticism or disbelief in the efficacy of medication may result in reduced levels of adherence.

Enhancing adherence

Evidence suggests that adequate counselling of patients in the use of their drugs can improve their adherence with the prescribed regimen. One study showed that intensive counselling by pharmacists of previously non-adherent hypertensive patients was effective in bringing about a significant improvement in adherence. However, on cessation of the counselling programme patients returned to their previously non-adherent behaviour (McKenney *et al.*, 1973).

The provision of simple comprehensive verbal instructions, devices to remind patients when to take their medicines, and the availability of patient information leaflets (PILs) may also be expected to enhance compliance. However, although PILs, which are a legal requirement for medicines, are a useful information source for medicine users there is no evidence that they have a significant effect on adherence (Raynor, 1992).

Patient adherence, like all illness behaviour, is influenced by factors such as social class, ethnic background, financial resources and the patient's level of education and understanding. An appreciation of how these factors influence health and illness behaviour will assist pharmacists in understanding the possible reasons for non-adherence, and may help in educating patients about medicines and the importance of adherence for their health. To achieve this, health professionals will need to communicate effectively with patients, and take into account the individual's personal and socio-economic circumstances.

In their study of pharmacists' health education activities, Shafford and Sharpe (1989) found that only a small minority of all enquiries made of pharmacists were related to general health matters, rather than directly to medicines. Such enquiries were predominantly concerned with weight loss, pregnancy, diet, smoking and family planning. The most frequent response to such enquiries was to give verbal advice, whilst information leaflets were provided as a response to 21 per cent of the consultations. Most consultations between pharmacists and patients relating to general health matters lasted between 5 and 10 minutes. Such a heavy demand on pharmacists' time additional to normal dispensing activities has serious implication if pharmacists are to significantly extend their activities into the health promotion arena. Such an expansion of pharmacists' activities, it has been argued, will necessitate the presence of more than one pharmacist in a pharmacy, or more likely changes in the way pharmacists supervise the dispensing of prescriptions, with routine work being carried out by accredited technical staff.

PHARMACY-BASED HEALTH PROMOTION

Health education and promotion form key elements of pharmacists' activities now and will become even more important in the future. As we have seen, pharmacists have a clear contribution to make in advising patients and the public on issues relating to minor illness and the use of purchased and prescribed medication, ensuring patient adherence. There is also potential for the provision of opportunistic community-based health education. Pharmacists' involvement in community based health promotion has expanded enormously in recent years. For instance, the introduction of 'high street' diagnostic testing and the availability of nicotine-replacement products have heightened the profile of the community pharmacy as a centre for health maintenance. Thus, community pharmacists can promote health on a range of issues, including those shown in Box 8.4.

There are many areas of health promotion in which pharmacists can have a significant input. These are described and discussed elsewhere (for instance, Blenkinsopp *et al.*, 2000; Harman, 2001). Here, we will consider in detail just one aspect of health promotion in which pharmacists would seem to have a particularly important role; namely, in addressing drug misuse. The term 'drug misuse' describes the misuse of purchased or prescribed medicines, and the use of illicit substances. Pharmacists may daily come into contact with people who are misusing a wide range of non-prescription medicines, such as laxatives. Pharmacists will also be aware of people who they suspect of dependence on prescribed medication.

For many years community pharmacists have supplied prescribed methadone to opiate drug misusers. Methadone maintenance therapy (MMT) aims to modify opiate misusers' habits, away from injection to oral consumption of methadone. Studies have indicated that the majority of pharmacists in the Birmingham Health Authority area (Jesson *et al.*, 2000) and the South East of England (Sheridan *et al.*, 1999) dispense methadone. In Scotland, 46 per cent of all community pharmacies dispense methadone, with the majority (65 per cent) of prescriptions being

---

Box 8.4 Issues about which pharmacists can offer advice and support (Blenkinsopp *et al.*, 2001)

- Smoking cessation
- Baby and child health
- Healthy eating
- Physical activity
- Drug misuse
- Contraception and sexual health
- Stress
- Oral health
- Accident prevention
- Prevention and early diagnosis of a range of diseases
- Promotion of screening and vaccination programmes

---

dispensed on a daily basis (Matheson *et al.*, 1999a). The expansion of methadone prescribing increases the risk of it entering or leaking into the illicit drug market, and hence the Advisory Council on the Misuse of Drugs (2000) has recommended that patients newly treated with methadone should have their consumption supervised for at least six months. However, community pharmacists themselves may not necessarily be prepared to provide such a service. A study of the attitudinal factors associated with the dispensing and supervision of consumption of methadone by community pharmacists in Scotland indicated a clear link between an individual pharmacist's attitudes and the provision of such services from the pharmacy (Matheson, 1999b).

In addition to dispensing methadone, community pharmacists have, over the past decade, played a key role in harm-minimisation strategies aimed at reducing the transfer of blood-borne viruses between injecting drug misusers. This has included programmes for the exchanges of injecting equipment and the sale of sterile injecting equipment. Whereas pharmacists' contract with the NHS requires them to supply methadone, if prescribed, they have no such obligation to either sell injecting equipment or to participate in a needle/syringe exchange scheme. Hence, in their contacts with drug misusers, community pharmacists may be more likely to dispense methadone on prescription than supply injecting equipment. Studies have shown that the provision of injecting equipment by pharmacists is more likely to occur when they have positive attitudes towards drug misusers (Rees *et al.*, 1997; Matheson *et al.*, 1999b).

The focus of drug policy today, then, has shifted away from the goal of abstinence and towards harm minimisation and, increasingly, decriminalisation. Pharmacists are among a range of health and social service personnel who are increasingly being brought into play to address the issue of drug misuse.

However, for pharmacists' contribution to have an impact in harm minimisation depends to a significant extent on their comprehension of the social context of health. This is equally important in all the other areas where pharmacists seek to engage in health-promoting activities. It is important to recognise that successful health promotion results in an impact on the public's health. The traditional didactic approach to health education has only a limited impact. Health promotion involves more than simply providing appropriate literature or standard verbal instructions to people. Health and illness behaviour is extraordinarily complex, and is influenced by a person's social environment. With an appreciation of the social processes associated with health and illness behaviour, pharmacists and health planners are more likely, and indeed more able, to develop health education programmes and health promotion that is more appropriate and effective in relation to the needs of the community.

SUMMARY

- Illness prevention is a major priority in health policy
- Health promotion is a key element of pharmacists' activities
- Multiple approaches to both health education and health promotion have been identified
- Pharmacists play an important part in ensuring that medicines are used appropriately.

FURTHER READING

Blenkinsopp, A., Panton, R.S. and Anderson, C. (2000) *Health Promotion for Pharmacists* (2nd edn), Oxford, Oxford University Press.

Downie, R.S., Tannahill, C. and Tannahill, A. (1996) *Health Promotion: Models and Values* (2nd edn), Oxford, Oxford University Press.

Harman, R.J. (ed.) (2001) *Handbook of Pharmacy Health Education* (2nd edn), London, Pharmaceutical Press.

REFERENCES

Acheson Report (1998) *Independent Inquiry into Inequalities in Health*, London, HMSO.

Advisory Council on the Misuse of Drugs (2000) *Reducing Drug Related Deaths: A Report of the Advisory Council on the Misuse of Drugs*, London, Stationery Office.

Anderson, C. (2000) Health Promotion in community pharmacy: the UK situation. *Patient Education and Counseling*, 39, 285–291.

Beattie, A. (1991) Knowledge and control in health promotion: a test case for social policy and social theory. In: J. Gabe, M. Calnan and M. Bury (eds) *The Sociology of the Health Service*, London, Routledge.

Bewley, B.R., Higgs, R.H. and Jones, A. (1984) Adolescent patients in an inner London general practice: their attitudes to illness and health care. *Journal of the Royal College of General Practitioners*, 34, 543–546.

Blenkinsopp, A., Anderson, C. and Panton, R. (2001) Promoting health. In: K.M.G. Taylor and G. Harding (eds) *Pharmacy Practice*, London, Taylor and Francis, pp. 151–164.

Blenkinsopp, A., Panton, R.S. and Anderson, C. (2000) *Health Promotion for Pharmacists* (2nd edn), Oxford, Oxford University Press.

Catford, J. and Nutbeam, D. (1984) Towards a definition of health education and health promotion. *Health Education Journal*, 43, 38.

Davison, C., Davey Smith, G. and Frankel, S. (1991) Lay epidemiology and the prevention paradox: the implications for coronary candidacy for health education. *Sociology of Health and Illness*, 13, 1–19.

Department of Health (1987) *Promoting Better Health*, London, HMSO.

Department of Health (1992) *The Health of the Nation: A Strategy for Health in England*, London, HMSO.

Department of Health (1996) *Primary Care: The Future*, London, HMSO.

Department of Health (1997) *The New NHS: Modern, Dependable*, London, Stationery Office.

Department of Health (1998) *Our Healthier Nation*, London, Stationery Office.

Department of Health (2000) *Pharmacy in the Future – Implementing the NHS Plan*, London, Department of Health.

Downie, R.S., Tannahill, C. and Tannahill, A. (1996) *Health Promotion: Models and Values* (2nd edn), Oxford, Oxford University Press.

Dunbar-Jacob, J.L., Dwyer, K. and Dunning, E.J. (1991) Compliance with anti-hypertensive regimen: a review of research in the 1980s. *Annals of Behavioural Medicine*, 13, 31–39.

Graham, H. (1984) *Women, Health and the Family*, Brighton, Wheatsheaf Books.

Harman, R.J. (ed.) (2001) *Handbook of Pharmacy Health Education* (2nd edn), London, Pharmaceutical Press.

Jesson, J., Wilson, K., Barton, A. and Pocock, R. (2000) Exploring the potential for supervised methadone consumption and shared care contracts with drug misusers. *Pharmaceutical Journal*, 265, R37.

Martin, C. and McQueen, D. (1989) Framework for a new public health. In: C. Martin and D. McQueen (eds) *Readings for a New Public Health*, Edinburgh, Edinburgh University Press.

Matheson, C., Bond, C.M. and Hickey, F. (1999a) Prescribing and dispensing for drug misusers in primary care: current practice in Scotland. *Family Practice*, 16, 375–379.

Matheson, C., Bond, C.M. and Mollison, J. (1999b) Attitudinal factors associated with community pharmacists' involvement in services for drug misusers. *Addiction*, 94, 1349–1359.

McClelland, C. and Rees, L. (2000) A foundation for health

promotion in pharmacy practice. In: P. Gard (ed.) *A Behavioural Approach to Pharmacy Practice*, Oxford, Blackwell Science.

McKenney, J.M., Slining, J.M., Henderson, H.R., Devins, D. and Barr, M. (1973) The effect of clinical pharmacy services on patients with essential hypertension. *Circulation*, 48, 1104–1111.

Nuffield Committee of Inquiry into Pharmacy (1986) *Pharmacy: A Report to the Nuffield Foundation*, London, Nuffield Foundation.

Petts, J. (2002) Health and local food initiatives. In: L. Adams, M. Amos and J. Munro (eds) *Promoting Health: Politics and Practice*, London, Sage.

Pharmaceutical Journal (1989) Compliance threat to first line asthma use. *Pharmaceutical Journal*, 243, 292.

Raynor, D.K. (1992) Patient compliance: the pharmacist's role. *International Journal of Pharmacy Practice*, 1, 126–135.

Rees, L., Harding, G. and Taylor, K.M.G. (1997) Supplying injecting equipment to drug misusers: a survey of community pharmacists' attitudes, beliefs and practices. *International Journal of Pharmacy Practice*, 5, 167–175.

Rodmell, S. and Watt, A. (1986) *The Politics of Health Education: Raising the Issues*, London, Routledge and Kegan Paul.

Royal Pharmaceutical Society of Great Britain (1996) *Pharmacy in a New Age: The New Horizon*, London, The Royal Pharmaceutical Society of Great Britain.

Royal Pharmaceutical Society of Great Britain (1997) *Pharmacy in a New Age: Building the Future*, London, The Royal Pharmaceutical Society of Great Britain.

Shafford, A. and Sharpe, K. (1989) *The Pharmacist as Health Educator*, London, Health Education Authority.

Sheridan, J., Strang, J. and Lovell, S. (1999) National and local guidance on services for drug misusers: do they influence current practice? – results of a survey of community pharmacists in South East England. *International Journal of Pharmacy Practice*, 7, 100–106.

Tannahill, A. (1985) What is health promotion? *Health Education Journal*, 44, 167–168.

Tones, B.K. (1986) Health education and the ideology of health promotion: a review of alternative approaches. *Health Education Research*, 1, 3–12.

Watt, A. (1986) Community Health Initiatives and their relationship to general practice. *Journal of the Royal College of General Practitioners*, 36, 72–73.

WHO (1996) *Good Pharmacy Practice (GPP) in Community and Hospital Pharmacy Settings*, WHO Document WHO/Pharm/DAP 96.1, Geneva, World Health Organisation.

WHO (1998) *Health 21: The Health for All Policy Framework for the WHO European Region*, European Health for All Series No. 5, Geneva, World Health Organisation.

9 Social Research Methods

INTRODUCTION

Research is becoming an increasingly important issue for all health care practitioners. This is epitomised by the increasing emphasis placed on evidence-based medicine (see Chapter 5). Indeed, the report of the Pharmacy Practice Research and Development Task Force (Royal Pharmaceutical Society of Great Britain,1997) stated: *'The whole of the [pharmacy] profession should be research-aware (i.e. research users) and a proportion should be research active (i.e. research doers).'*

Consequently, it is essential that all pharmacists have an understanding of the methodologies underpinning research and are able to interpret, evaluate and apply research findings. In this chapter we focus on social research methods which are widely used in pharmacy practice and health services research.

As highlighted throughout the previous chapters, social action is complex and consequently its study requires specific and appropriate methodologies. As with all research, social research must be rigorous and involves the use of appropriate methodological tools to address specific research questions. Because of the nature of social research, it is frequently necessary to secure prior approval of the research from the appropriate Ethics Committee, and sufficient time should be allowed for this when planning such research.

When carrying out research a series of choices are made in response to some preliminary questions. These questions which should be asked at the early stage of any research include:

- What is the area of study or investigation?
- What type of question or problem is the research aiming to address?
- What research design is most appropriate to this research question?
- What would be the most appropriate method or methods?
- What would be the most relevant research tools?

The most difficult, and yet most crucial aspect of any research is asking the right question. The form of that question in turn will influence the research methods and techniques later employed. For example, if we were asking a 'how many?' or 'how often?' type of question – for instance: how frequently do pharmacists communicate directly with general practitioners? – then a survey would be appropriate. If, however, we wanted to study in more detail the nature of communication and interaction between pharmacists and general practitioners, we might undertake direct observation techniques or use depth interviews.

For researchers working within the disciplines of the natural sciences the choice of research strategy is governed by the assumptions of the scientific community. One feature of the natural scientist's activities is that they are dealing with material objects – for example, a chemical structure or a human organ. Moreover, it is assumed that by routine, systematic observation and by careful recording of data, knowledge of the interrelation between material objects is accumulated: as, for instance, in the discovery and study of the pharmacological actions of a drug on the body, or the study of the physicochemical properties of a drug compound. This direct, observational approach is known as empiricism or an empirical approach. The properties of materials are thus understood and classified, and this classification provides scientists with models with which to understand the actions and properties of similar materials. These models are therefore inextricably linked to the methods that are used to build them. That is to say, the assumptions we hold about materials determine our choice of the methodological tools which we employ to investigate them.

The link between our assumptions and our methods of analysis is perhaps a less contentious issue amongst natural scientists than among social scientists. This is because social scientists do not necessarily share a common set of assumptions about individuals' social behaviour. Consequently, there is not one single method of social research, but several, each of which assumes a particular theoretical model of social behaviour. However, irrespective of whether research is in the natural or social sciences, Shipman (1988) suggests four key questions should be addressed when conducting research. They are:

1. If the investigation were to be carried out again, by different researchers, using the same methods, would the same results be obtained?
2. Does the evidence reflect the reality under investigation?
3. What relevance do the results have beyond the situation investigated?
4. Is there sufficient detail on the way the evidence was produced for the credibility of the research to be assessed?

Only by making clear the researcher's assumptions about social behaviour, which are implicit in the research methodology, will these questions be adequately addressed. Shipman's key questions provide a useful starting point from which to consider the approach the research is to take, but, while all these questions are appropriate to quantitative approaches to research, it is important to remember that qualitative social research methods are based on interpretation of the data by the researcher, and as such different researchers may bring different perspectives to the same data.

The experimental method

The randomised controlled trial (RCT) is established as the 'gold standard' of empirical, clinical research and is widely used as an experimental tool. The RCT is not specifically addressed here as this methodology is largely a clinical rather than social research tool. Within social research, the experimental method implies that the researcher intervenes in a process, the effects of which are then observed and measured. It concerns the attempt to control all the variables affecting that which is being studied, the aim being to try and identify causal relationships. Something about the social action in question is being measured. Researchers begin this type of research by developing theoretical models about the way individuals act under given circumstances; they carry out experiments to test these predictions. To illustrate, it could be hypothesised that the use of fluoride toothpaste will affect the rate of tooth decay in children. Two groups of children would be selected, being matched for age, sex, social class, height, schooling etc. and given a dental inspection. The experimental group are provided with a year's supply of fluoride toothpaste, the control group with ordinary toothpaste. After one year a post-test dental examination finds that the experimental group have significantly less decay. The researchers would then draw conclusions on the basis of this observation.

Methods of social analysis

Social research methods can be classified as being either qualitative or quantitative. Though such categories are not mutually exclusive, we shall use this dichotomy to organise the material in this chapter. These divergent approaches adopt different research tools and are based upon, and informed by, different theoretical foundations. The dichotomy is not always clear-cut, and both quantitative and qualitative methods can be used together; they yield different types of data, and the one may well complement the other. Within these two approaches there are many types of research methods.

Sampling strategies

The choice of sampling strategy will be determined by the type of methodology used. With quantitative methods, the sampling strategies are designed to ensure that the results will be both valid and generalisable (probability sampling). Qualitative methods, however, use different sampling strategies (non-probability sampling).

The most rigorously constructed survey schedule can yield consistently biased data if it is not applied to a representative sample of the population being surveyed. The most elementary sampling technique – selecting a specific number of respondents at random, is no less problematic than more sophisticated procedures such as stratified sampling. This is because sampling, by its nature, always involves an element of bias and error. The principle underlying random sampling is that each unit within the population surveyed has an equal chance of being selected. To illustrate, a random sample of ten pieces of coal selected from a mound would involve more than making a selection from the pieces of coal immediately to hand. The heavier pieces would be more likely to be at the bottom of the pile than the top; pieces in the centre of the pile would be excluded from being selected because they would not be immediately accessible, and so forth. Strictly speaking there is no such thing as a truly 'random sample'. When attempting to draw up a random sample, then, every attempt must be made to ensure that the elements comprising the population, from which the sample is to be taken, whether the sample comprises lumps of coal or patients presenting to a pharmacist, have an equal chance of being selected. For this purpose random number tables, which are frequently published in statistical textbooks, may be used as a means of drawing up a random sample.

The decision whether or not to sample, and the choice of sampling techniques, will be determined not least by the cost of conducting a survey and the demand for accuracy and precision. Only by surveying the total population can the optimum degree of precision be guaranteed. While this may be a viable option for surveys of very small populations, more often the cost of administering the survey to a total population will be prohibitive. A sample will therefore have to be taken.

Two popular methods of probability sampling are:

1. *Simple random sample* – involves a random selection of a specific number of units drawn from the population investigated which is treated as an undifferentiated whole.
2. *Stratified random sample* – involves breaking the investigated population into distinct sub-groups or strata, and then randomly selecting a specific number of units from each stratum.

Three sampling strategies for qualitative research are:

1. *Maximum variety sampling* – purposively selecting individuals by certain criteria relevant to the research in order to solicit as wide a range of experiences as possible.
2. *Convenience sampling* – selecting individuals who are available in the study context. For example, identifying individuals for

inclusion in a study by their attendance at a pharmacy on a particular day.

3. *Theoretic sampling* – purposively selecting individuals by criteria relevant to the theory being explored. For example, an investigation into the public's perception of pharmacy as a retail outlet might be informed by the theoretical construct of the public as health care consumers rather than patients. A theoretic sampling might therefore involve selecting individuals considered to explore this theory.

A considerable amount has been written about both the theory and techniques of survey sampling; further details can be found in the texts recommended at the end of this chapter.

QUANTITATIVE RESEARCH METHODS

The purpose of quantitative methods is to generate precise measurements of social action, which can be explained by the aggregation of statistical data.

Quantitative research aims to:

1. Explain social behaviour in terms of a cause and effect relationship, with the social action as the effect and an underlying governing principle the cause – for example, it may be argued that juvenile delinquency is caused by poverty.
2. Measure social behaviour by objective criteria – for example, how often a patient consults a pharmacist (a consultation being defined in a set of objective criteria, not as defined by either the patient or the pharmacist).

The experimental method is often used as the organising principle of quantitative research.

Social surveys

Surveys are a means of collecting information from large samples of the population relatively quickly and efficiently, and allow comparisons to be made between individuals and groups. Conducting a survey requires that the researcher pays particular attention to its design. For instance, it would be necessary to ensure that a representative sample is drawn, and that the survey is organised adequately – that is, that the questionnaire schedule is appropriate and that researchers are suitably trained.

Social survey interviews involve a structured dialogue – the questions are pre-formulated in order to elicit specific answers. These answers form the social survey data. Success in obtaining the required data depends on asking the appropriate questions.

There are two principal considerations to be borne in mind when designing survey questions:

1. The question must be clearly intelligible to the respondent.
2. Care should be taken to ensure that all respondents could provide an appropriate answer to the question.

Textbooks which provide information on how to phrase questions are available on survey research methods. Whilst the subject of the survey and the population to be surveyed will govern the nature of the questions, there are several precepts to be applied when phrasing survey questions. Survey research aims to elicit responses based on a series of specific questions. An ambiguous question may produce an answer based on an idiosyncratic interpretation by the respondent. Such data is unacceptable because the answers would not be comparable. Technical language has a precise meaning and should be used only if the survey population could be expected to be familiar with it. Otherwise jargon should be avoided as inappropriate. Clarity is important since there is less likelihood that the question will be misinterpreted; however, patronising phrasing should be avoided. Questions to which there is a wide range of possible responses, or which combine a number of questions into one, are often difficult to answer, and the responses are even more difficult to analyse. One solution is to provide a checklist of possible responses to a single question together with instruction on the number of responses to be entered. Negatively phrased questions and questions requiring detailed recall by respondents do little to promote accurate answers.

The survey method produces invaluable data for social scientists but may suffer from being superficial in the sense that it cannot always glean the more subtle aspects of human behaviour.

Self-completed questionnaire design

The correct phrasing of survey questions is particularly crucial in the design of a self-completed questionnaire. Questions designed to elicit the attitudes and values of respondents are not likely to produce adequate answers. The reasons for holding particular attitudes and values are often very complex, and cannot be adequately represented from responses to pre-formulated questions. For this reason, many self-completed questionnaires are comprised of a series of 'closed' questions; that is to say, questions having a very restricted range of possible responses – for example, 'Have you used this pharmacy before?' To such a question the respondent can only answer 'Yes', 'No' or 'Don't know'. Closed questions have the virtue of being easy to answer by the respondent and are relatively simple to analyse.

While the general nature of the questions to be asked will be determined by the subject of the survey, the actual selection of questions should be generated from preliminary studies of the population to be surveyed. Before planning specific questions it is important to establish the possible scope of the issues to be surveyed. This may involve unstructured interviews with a small sample from the proposed survey population. Additional background information may be obtained from a variety of other sources, including previous survey data. The importance of this preliminary work cannot be overstated. Self-completed questionnaire surveys are an unsolicited intrusion on the survey population. It is crucial that the information sought cannot be readily obtained from other sources, and that it will achieve the survey's objective.

Once the questions have been compiled the completed questionnaire should be 'piloted'. This usually involves administering the questionnaire to a small sample of respondents. The returned questionnaires will highlight any inadequacies in the questionnaire's content and wording, and may indicate any potential difficulties with analysis of the full survey data.

Response rates

A postal self-completed questionnaire is effectively unsolicited mail and may be treated as such by the recipient. The success of the survey therefore relies on eliciting the co-operation of the respondent in completing and returning the questionnaire. A number of measures may facilitate an acceptable response rate (Box 9.1).

It is very important to have a strategy for following up non-respondents (those unable or unwilling to reply) to a postal questionnaire survey. At least one reminder should be issued to non-respondents. Further reminders may be issued to persistent non-respondents but are likely to have a markedly more reduced effect than the first. An alternative to the second reminder, if at all feasible, is to contact the non-respondent by telephone. A

Box 9.1 Strategies to ensure an acceptable response rate for postal questionnaires

1. Enclose a stamped addressed envelope
2. Personalise the introductory letter
3. Clearly print the questionnaire
4. Ensure the relevance of the questionnaire to the respondent
5. Secure prior approval from any appropriate official body, such as an Ethics Committee
6. Register the data in accordance with the Data Protection Act
7. Stress confidentiality of the data and anonymity of the respondent
8. Prior announcement of the study in the appropriate journals
9. Offer some kind of incentive, such as a free sachet of coffee or entry into a draw for a free day's locum

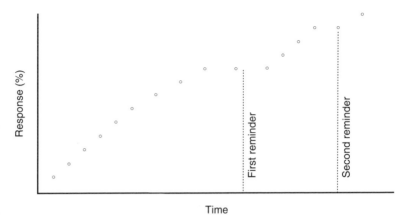

Figure 9.1 Effect of reminders on the response rate of self-completed questionnaire surveys

telephone call has the advantage of establishing whether the postal questionnaire was ever received, and whether the respondent actually intends to complete and return the questionnaire. The timing for any strategy for issuing reminders is equally important – if issued too early, potential respondents may feel pestered, but if issued too late this may indicate to the respondent the survey's lack of urgency (and possibly its lack of importance) (see Figure 9.1).

It has been reported that the response rate achieved in published survey research among community pharmacists ranges from 20–90 per cent, with approximately one-third less than 50 per cent and one-third greater than 70 per cent (Smith, 2002). In studies where the response rate is low, and where there is no apparent attempt to investigate non-responders, the sample effectively becomes self-selecting and the findings can only be speculatively generalised beyond that sample (Smith, 2002).

Survey question form and content

Surveys have become a particularly popular method of social research, possibly because of their apparent simplicity. Essentially, social surveys involve a researcher administering pre-formulated questions to a number of potential respondents. Administering a social survey is indeed relatively straightforward, but the amount and quality of information obtained requires considerable preliminary work prior to administrating the survey if useful and usable data is to be obtained.

There are several mistakes to avoid in the difficult task of constructing survey questions. The suggestions below are not exhaustive, nor are the potential errors indicated necessarily mutually exclusive; however, it is hoped these will indicate some of the more obvious pitfalls, which with careful planning can be avoided.

1. Inappropriate question form
It is important to choose the appropriate form of question (closed or open) to elicit the response desired:

'Do you have opinions on . . .?' (closed)
'What are your opinions on . . .?' (open)

In this example a closed question is an inappropriate form to elicit an opinion. The obvious answer to the closed question is either 'Yes' or 'No'. Both these answers reveal nothing of the actual opinions held.

2. Loaded or leading questions
Implicit in these types of question is the desired or expected answer. An example of a loaded question might be:

'Do you, like most other pharmacists, consider that the Royal Pharmaceutical Society's "Pharmacy in a New Age" campaign was a success?'

A leading question may produce more information than a loaded question, though it may not necessarily reflect accurately the individual's true response. For example:

'Following the Crown Report on supplementary prescribing, do you think the pharmacist should be involved in prescribing medicines for patients?'

3. Two questions in one
In this case, no simple answer is possible. For instance:

'Does having a pharmacy within the health centre make querying a prescription with the prescriber easier; has this benefited patients?'

'Do you think aspirin and paracetamol are appropriate treatments for migraine?'

4. Double negative
The answer, 'Yes' or 'No', to such questions may not convey what the respondent actually believed. For instance:

'Do you consider not contacting the prescriber about a potential drug interaction on a prescription is unprofessional?'

And taking things to extremes:

'Do you not think that not continuing to take a prescribed

antibiotic, until the course is completed, is an inappropriate response to failure of the medication.'

5. *Complex questions*
Similarly, complex questions may not permit the respondent to reveal their true beliefs. For instance:

> 'If doctors are going to be held responsible for their own budgets do you believe that pharmacists, with their knowledge of drug costs, should have a more interactive role with prescribers at the point when a prescription is written, or not.'

6. *Abbreviations, jargon or technical language*
Examples:

> 'Do you keep PMRs in this pharmacy?'

> 'Do you think the introduction of compulsory CPD will enhance the professional standing of pharmacists?'

Abbreviations such as 'PMR' and 'CPD' may be confusing to the respondents, and consequently the benefits of using abbreviations to shorten the length of the question are outweighed by the risks of eliciting a confused or inappropriate response. Similarly, with the question:

> 'After inhaling your bronchodilator aerosol do you hold your breath for ten seconds before exhaling?'

Terms such as 'inhaling' and 'exhaling' may not be readily understood by respondents not acquainted with medical terminology. The question loses nothing by replacing these words with 'breathing in' and 'breathing out'. The word 'bronchodilator' could be omitted altogether, or if appropriate replaced with 'reliever'. Similar confusion may arise over the use of such terms as 'fracture', 'prophylactic', 'topical', 'gastro-intestinal', 'regimen', etc.

7. *Conversational*
Questions such as:

> 'How do you find you get on with the general practitioners?'

> 'Do you employ a general assistant to help out in the dispensary?'

In these examples 'get on' and 'help out' are not defined. The answers to these questions will not be comparable because respondents do not have a shared definition.

8. *Ambiguous questions*

'How long has the pharmacy been open?'

Though the question is clearly designed to establish the duration in months and years, the question may invite the facetious answer: 'Since 8.30 this morning, as usual!'

Another commonly encountered type of ambiguity is contained in the question:

'How long have you worked in this pharmacy?
0–5 years
5–10 years
10–20 years
20 years or more

The question clearly poses a problem for respondents for whom the answer is 5, 10 or 20 years.

9. *Vagueness and imprecision*
Consider a question such as:

'How long have you been a pharmacist?'

This will elicit useful information, but by careful forethought more detailed or precise information could be obtained, by for instance asking:

'When did you first register as a pharmacist?' or

'How long have you worked full-time (i.e. 30 hours or more per week) in this pharmacy?'

The following question is similarly flawed:

'How frequently do you (the pharmacist) and local general practitioners consult with each other?'

The response to this question will simply be an estimate of the sum total of all consultations between pharmacist and general practitioners. It will provide no information as to who initiated the consultation.

10. *Hypothetical questions*
It is important from the outset that it is realised that such questions can only elicit attitudes and opinions, not factual information. For instance:

'Do you think pharmacists should have access to patient medication records held by the prescriber?'

11. *Meaningless or inappropriate questions*

> 'Is the *Pharmaceutical Journal* as good as the *Chemist and Druggist?'*

The aims and content of the two publications are completely different and therefore one is not an appropriate alternative to the other.

Data processing

Computer programs designed to process survey data have developed rapidly in recent years and those such as the Statistical Package for the Social Science (SPSS) are relatively simple to master and designed specifically to handle social survey data.

Computer processing of survey data requires each of the responses to the survey to be assigned an individual code. The techniques for coding survey questions are covered comprehensively in the literature outlined in the Further Reading section at the end of this chapter, and recent software developments have made the process of entering coded data relatively straightforward. Moreover, these programs can perform a myriad of statistical analyses on the data, but ultimately it is up to the researcher to make sense of the findings. The sheer complexity and power of these programs can be seductive, and a range of statistical tests may be applied to the data simply because they are available. Often such a plethora of results may be a hindrance rather than a help in making sense of the data. For this reason it is useful to decide, when planning the survey, what statistical tests are necessary to meet the survey's objectives.

Data Protection Act

Researchers using a computer to store details of any living person are required to register with the Data Protection Registrar, in accordance with the Data Protection Act (1998). Although the majority of institutions holding computer records of their personnel are already registered, if the institution wishes to obtain data for research purposes, details of the information to be collected, together with those who will obtain it, are required to be registered with the Data Protection Registrar. Registration requires that the data collected must comply with eight principles of good practice (Box 9.2).

Box 9.2 Principles of good data collection practice

Analysis of quantitative data

Having collected quantitative data, most often in the form of completed postal questionnaires, and entered this for processing by computer, the results obtained require analysis. This involves the application of statistical tests. Selected texts on the application of statistical tests are given at the end of this chapter. The concern here is with the underlying principles of quantitative analysis.

Statistical tests are used to establish whether the overall picture presented by the data occurred because of an *actual* underlying association or relationship within the data, or whether the relationship is merely a chance phenomenon. To determine the nature of this relationship the significance of the statistical relationship has to be determined.

For example, if we examined a sample of adult patients attending a pharmacy in a single day and discovered the ratio of women to men was 10:1 we would not conclude that women had a tenfold greater rate of visiting pharmacies compared with men. Reproducing the study on the following day may reveal a ratio of 6:1. Having replicated the study many times over, and determining the mean of all the observations, we may find the ratio of 7:1. The question is, was the observed data a reflection of the actual ratio of women to men, or was the ratio of 7:1 merely due to chance? Statistical tests are therefore applied to data to estimate the extent to which chance played a part in determining the data collected. Key to these statistical tests is the concept of probability.

What is probability?

Probability in the statistical sense is a measure indicating the likelihood of an event happening – most usually these events in clinical research describe a relationship or association between two or more events. Probability is expressed as a decimal fraction – thus when throwing a dice there is a one-in-six chance of a six coming up. This is expressed statistically as 0.167. Should our dice be marked with two sixes, the probability of rolling a six increases to 0.334, and so on. The greater the measure of probability, the less likely our recorded data can be attributed to chance alone, i.e. it indicates an actual rather than chance relationship or association.

Measuring probability

Applying probability in statistical tests is less straightforward than might be expected. Consider, for example, a study of two types of treatment for depression where one appears more effective than another. The analysis of the results commences with the hypothesis that the difference observed is down to chance alone and that in actuality there is no difference between the two. This, rather pessimistically, is termed the 'null hypothesis' call. As we can never account for every single possible factor whose influence may contribute to the observed difference, the only valid assumption we can proceed from is that the play of chance accounts for the observed difference. Statistical tests then calculate the likelihood of the observed or greater difference occurring by chance alone, which is expressed as a level of probability or P value. The smaller the P value the greater our conviction that the observed differences are less likely to be due to chance alone. Therefore if the P value from the study comparing the two different treatments is very small, i.e. $P = 0.001$ (i.e. there is a 1 in 1,000 probability that the result is due to chance) it may be concluded that the results of the comparison are not due to chance. In doing so we would reject the null hypothesis and consider the observed difference to be other than a chance event.

The question then is when is a P value small enough to allow rejection of the null hypothesis? Conventionally, a P value which is less than 0.05 or $P < 0.05$ is widely regarded as allowing us to reject chance as accounting for an observed difference. P values of < 0.05 thus allow the observed difference to have achieved what is termed statistical significance.

Confidence intervals

An alternative method for assessing the effects of chance on observed differences is to consider confidence intervals. Unlike the calculated P value, which only indicates whether the observed difference may in fact be the effect of chance, confidence limits indicate how small or large the actual size of the effect of chance might be on the observed differences.

In order to establish whether the observed difference is influenced by chance we need to establish whether the actual difference could be as low as zero – that is, there is no actual difference, and that the observed difference is attributed to chance. To do so we usually need to establish the range within which we can be 95 per cent certain the actual value lies. If, for example, a clinical trial of two drugs for depression produces an average difference of 5, on a scale for measuring levels of depression, this value could be influenced by chance. We therefore need to establish whether the actual value for the difference in the two treatments could be zero – that is, there is no difference between the two treatments. If the confidence intervals at the 95 per cent level were between, say, 3 and 8 we could say that the observed difference has a P value of $P < 0.05$ and was thus statistically significant. Should there be a wider confidence interval of, say, -3 to 16 then the actual value could include zero, in which case we would conclude that there was no significant difference between the effects of the two drugs. Confidence intervals therefore show how small and how large are the effects of chance, whereas P values only indicate whether the result might be an effect of chance.

Reliability, validity and causality

The reliability and validity of accumulated data are fundamental to good research.

Reliability concerns the extent to which measurements, if repeated under the same conditions, yield the same results. For example, if a standardised interview was administered by different interviewers the same results should be produced.

Validity refers to the extent to which the research instruments or measures, measure what they purport to measure. Quite clearly the extent to which one's research results are valid is of paramount importance.

It is important to note that reliability and validity are not necessarily synonymous. For example, an intelligence test may be reliable in that it produces consistent results, but it may not be measuring intelligence as was understood in the research hypothesis, and as such the results may be invalid. There are many different types of validity (Cook and Campbell, 1979). It is important to distinguish between *internal* and *external* validity.

Internal validity concerns whether the research method employed is actually measuring the phenomenon being investigated. *External validity* concerns the extent to which the research results can be generalised beyond the population studied. For instance, a survey of people's attitudes to pharmacies, conducted within pharmacies, may be 'self-selecting' in that only the attitudes of those people who visit a pharmacy will be measured, and the attitudes of those who don't will be excluded. One strategy to enhance the level of external validity in survey research involves sampling procedures. The main sampling strategies have been discussed above.

Experimental and survey research involves a process of ruling out plausible alternative explanations, such that *'the only process available for establishing a scientific theory is one of eliminating plausible rival hypothesis'* (Cook and Campbell, 1979). This is what the philosopher, Karl Popper (1902–94) termed 'falsification' or the 'hypothetico-deductive method'. The hypothetico-deductive method involves first establishing a hypothesis, drawn from interviews, observations and such like, which could be refuted empirically; that is, it is 'testable'. If a hypothesis continues to hold, despite experiments designed to disprove it, it becomes accepted as a 'deductive causal' explanation, though not as proof. To illustrate this point, Popper used the example of a swan. We may wish to hypothesise that all swans are white. To test this hypothesis empirically we may conduct an exhaustive search of many swans and find, without exception, that all swans we have observed are indeed white. Our findings therefore allow the hypothesis to stand. However, we have not proved all swans are white, only that we have been unable to refute the hypothesis. The discovery of a single black swan would be sufficient to reject the hypothesis.

The implications for research which relies exclusively on statistics are considerable. For example, statistical correlations, based on the types of surveys we have described, in many ways provide the starting point for the development of theories and explanations. Social research involves trying to 'explain' these findings – for instance, that ill-health is significantly (statistically) associated with poverty. However, it is crucial not to get carried away with statistical relationships, for it is all too easy to fall into the trap of making 'invalid' assumptions about the relationship between two variables. Researchers usually seek to understand the causal connections between variables which change simultaneously.

To illustrate this, variable A (excessive consumption of animal fats) may be associated with variable B (heart disease). In a study we want to elicit which variable is 'responsible' or 'independent' and which is 'dependent'. We need to be certain which is the independent and which is the dependent variable – that is, does A cause B or B cause A. If we were to say that A (excessive consumption of animal fats) was the independent variable and B (heart disease) was the dependent variable, we would need to meet at least three basic criteria to ensure that this statement was valid:

1. *Correlation:* an association between two variables must be statistically significant. For instance, self-esteem may be found to vary with educational achievement.
2. *Time:* we must be sure that the independent variable occurs prior to the dependent variable. For instance, did the school child feel a failure because she failed her exams or did she fail her exams because she felt a failure? Such problems could easily confound a study of educational achievement, especially if the study was retrospective.
3. *Extraneous factors:* that is, variables which may affect both A and B. For instance, poor educational achievement (B) may be associated with a child's low self-esteem (A), but may also be associated with other factors, such as poor housing (X)

The point we are trying to highlight here is that to create a 'causal model' is an extremely precarious process in social research and it is always to a greater or lesser extent circumscribed because:

1. it is impossible to set up an experiment with water-tight control groups, and
2. in social research we are dealing with human beings whose actions, unlike the actions of chemicals, are influenced by how they make sense of their surroundings and their interpretations of happenings around them.

Another problem in establishing causal models to understand the social world is the multiplicity of factors involved in social processes; for example, there are many social factors (outlined in Chapter 5) which affect people's health.

QUALITATIVE RESEARCH METHODS

Many 'real life' situations do not lend themselves to investigation by precise statistical measurement, and cannot be fully understood by the aggregation of statistical data. Qualitative research, by way of direct observation and involvement with people under study, aims for a detailed description and understanding of what people really think, how they structure and organise their thoughts, from where they derive their ideas and how they are likely to act in particular circumstances. The emphasis is on naturally occurring events rather than on the aggregation of observations of a series of behaviours, views or attitudes. The aim of such research is to facilitate an in-depth understanding and an appreciation of the meanings people attach to what they do or believe. Qualitative research aims to elicit:

1. What people 'really think', from where they derive their ideas and beliefs, how they organise and structure their ideas.
2. How people act in their 'natural' settings.
3. Social action as it occurs. Unlike in the laboratory it is often unrealistic or impossible to create experimental conditions to control for all, if any, of the extraneous variables – for example, it would be virtually impossible to study behaviour at football matches in such a 'controlled' way.

The main research tools of qualitative analyses are:

1. *Participant observation* – the observer participates in the daily lives of people under study, observing things that happen and listening to what is said, and then makes notes of his or her observation. For example, a researcher, trained as a consultant

in OTC drug information, worked in a community pharmacy as a member of staff and was able to collect data relating to the need for and uptake of information relating to the purchase of medicines (Nichol *et al.*, 1992).

2. *Group interviews/discussions* – the researcher, with the aid of a list of relevant topics, guides the conversation among a small group of respondents. Often, the researcher will pursue subjects which emerge spontaneously as well as the pre-defined topics. The interaction between members of the group is an essential component of a methodology, which may also be referred to as focus groups. For instance, Jesson *et al.* (1994) employed focus group discussions as one of a range of research tools to investigate consumers' perceptions of pharmacy health education literature. The group discussions were used in order to explore the key issues of importance to consumers and from this to formulate a research agenda from the consumers' perspective.

3. *Semi-structured or conversational interviews.* Unlike questionnaires, where the questions are predetermined and uniform to allow for the aggregation of responses, the interviewer talks with the respondent informally around the topics relevant to his or her research. With the aid of a list of topics the interviewer pursues subjects as they arise and follows relevant leads. The role of the interviewer is non-directive and yet not wholly passive, because he or she must assess how what is being said relates to the research focus. Interviewing requires a great deal of skill and therefore the interviewer should be trained so that they possess the necessary qualities. For instance, depth interviews, using a topic guide to direct the interview, have produced a great deal of the data on people's beliefs and conceptualisations of health and illness (see Chapter 4). They have also been used extensively to explore issues relating to pharmaceutical service delivery and professional practice from the viewpoint of pharmacists and the public.

Qualitative research is usually small scale and aims at eliciting a richness of detail rather than statistical generalisations. That is, we can learn a great deal about a particular social situation, or how people interact with each other in given situations, but we cannot make claims that the findings would hold true beyond our field of study (i.e. they are not generalisable). Social science has also gained from 'case study' research which often, although not exclusively, uses qualitative research methods. By 'case study' we mean the detailed examination of a single example or case (for instance, a small society, a pharmacy, an organisation, or a health centre). For comparative purposes, a series of case studies may be undertaken.

One of the main advantages of this type of research is that we are able to see people within their natural context. Sociologists, and in particular medical sociologists, have in recent years increasingly come to appreciate the value of being able to relate what people say and do to their individual circumstances.

Participant observation and ethnographic research

Participant observation, as the name implies, involves fully participating among those being studied. For example, to understand the impact of pharmacy-based methadone supervision on drug misuse the researcher might operate as a counter assistant to obtain observational data. More likely, however, the method may be adapted to involve the researcher passively watching, listening, keeping diaries, or examining records.

Ethnographic research assumes the importance of people's perspectives, perceptions and actions, and the meanings they attribute to these. People's views, beliefs and actions are observed within the context of their everyday lives. The philosophy underlying the ethnographic approach diverges from traditional survey research. The latter is closely allied to the natural sciences in that it is characterised by testing models and hypotheses. Ethnographic research has no clearly defined hypothesis to be tested; instead data, rather than being discovered, are uncovered. Data collection is an exploratory process; it is 'inductive' rather than 'deductive' reasoning which is inherent in such experimental studies.

Interviews

One of the most common forms of data collection in social research is the interview. Much has been written on the nature, types and pitfalls of the interview. A brief introduction is provided here.

Standardised or structured interviews

These involve eliciting the same information from every respondent. The questions must be designed to ensure that the answers are comparable and classifiable. There are two forms of standardised interviews:

- *Scheduled interviews*, where the wording and sequence of questions are determined in advance and questions are asked in the same way.
- *Non-schedule interviews*, where the questions may be asked in any order, as is considered appropriate by the interviewer during the interview. In this case the interviewer is told the information required and is allowed to vary the order and nature of questions if appropriate.

Non-standardised, depth interviews

These may take many forms, but the interviewer is not restricted to pre-set questions as there is no attempt to gain the same classifiable categories of information from every respondent. Such an interview may take the form of specific open questions or merely a list of topics to be discussed. There are three important characteristics of this method:

- Flexibility – the interviewer must be able to adapt and respond to the individual and their circumstances.
- Responsive or interactive – the interviewer must keep alert to pursue interesting ideas or 'leads'.
- Probing – the interviewer must pursue the respondent's initial reasoning by asking further questions.

This type of interviewing requires a considerable degree of skill and expertise, and it is essential that interviewers are suitably trained for this task.

Analysis of qualitative data

Analysis using grounded theory

In direct contrast to the construction of a hypothesis for testing is an alternative approach, which starts with no predefined ideas or theories, instead allowing theories to emerge from the data. This is referred to as 'grounded theory' (Glaser and Strauss, 1967). Collected data are fitted into categories, and subsequent data are then amassed to establish the veracity of these categories and develop others. These categories are then used to formulate theory. This approach is, however, deceptively simple, as a theory grounded in the data is necessarily not generated in abstraction from the social world but from an *a priori* appreciation of the relationship between the data collected, through observations and interviews, and its social context.

Analysis using sociological theory

Reference to textbooks detailing methods of analysing qualitative data are to be found at the end of this chapter. With many texts designed for those conducting 'applied research' – that is, research addressing practical issues rather than so-called 'pure research', which explores issues within the framework of a particular discipline (e.g. psychology, anthropology and sociology) – the novice qualitative researcher is frequently 'faced with a smorgasbord of methods' (Baum, 1995). In such texts, the technical applications of qualitative methods are spelled out as formulae, or computer software programs as a means of exploring how people make sense of their world, and to generate insights into people's health-related behaviour not readily accessible through surveys.

Most often, the application of a qualitative analysis involves methods for extracting themes from transcripts of interviews. Such approaches, however, run the risk of generating qualitative insights that may differ little from common sense. This is because such formulaic approaches are often founded on the principles of what the leading American Sociologist Mills, in his critique of the atheoretical nature of much qualitative research, termed 'abstracted empiricism' (Mills, 1959). The 'insights' from the research are frequently presented as quotes derived by researchers from interviews and as such are shallow. That is, the data is assumed to speak for itself and that 'analysis' is simply a question of organising the data into themes – for which it is not necessary to understand the underlying assumptions behind the method.

Problem-oriented qualitative analysis, which seeks to address a specific 'practical' research problem, such as how to contain pre-scribing costs or how to identify the constituent elements of 'best practice', is generally concerned with the assembly of 'facts' and descriptions. The scope of problem-oriented qualitative research questions, and the chosen method of analysis, becomes defined, then, by practical rather than theoretical considerations. Tran-scripts and notes recounting experiences, views, and beliefs are assumed to be empirically self-evident. Problem-oriented quali-tative research thus becomes little more than a set of simple tech-niques or practices as in 'content analysis' (Krippendorff, 1980), which involves identifying and cataloguing themes from tran-scripts.

To treat what people say and do as self-evident reduces the power of qualitative analysis to little more than accumulated accounts of common sense. In turn this leads to the discrete accu-mulation of empirical data. Yet qualitative analysis should extend beyond ordering the content of individuals' responses and narra-tives along identified themes. The question becomes not simply what pattern can be discerned from people's narratives but also why this pattern and not others? The task when undertaking a qualitative analysis requires the researcher to approach the task with searching and penetrating questions – not simply gathering together recurrent issues into arbitrary themes. Although many factors should be considered, from our collective experience we believe the following key pointers can serve as a guide to conduct-ing rigorous qualitative analysis of transcripts.

1. *Transcripts should be analysed, not simply presented as descriptive anecdotes*
Many published qualitative studies based on depth interviews

share a similar presentational format. That is, the raw data (i.e. selected quotes) are grouped together, and listed according to identified themes, to generate an explanatory account of individuals' actions. For instance, whilst it is interesting and informative to learn from a series of quotes that the majority of community pharmacists do not believe that it is in their interests to offer blood-cholesterol testing in their pharmacies, the real value of a qualitative analysis is in exploring *why* this is the case.

2. *Interview transcripts are public accounts*

A popular methodological tool for qualitative researchers is the depth interview. Accessing authentic details of how people account for their actions, their beliefs and behaviour, however, is an accomplishment requiring skill in both interviewing and analysing interview data. Interviews can be (and frequently are) unsolicited and occasionally intrusive social encounters. As such, the relationship between interviewer and interviewee is necessarily artificial. For instance, one would not expect to find the sort of formal verbal exchange characteristic of interviews taking place in a pub or workplace between close associates, friends or colleagues. The very nature of the interview process itself thus often commences with the interviewer and interviewee adopting a rather stilted posture in relation to what is said and how it is said. That is to say, the answers provided by the interviewee will, in the first instance, be sanitised – no one is going to reveal what they really feel (they may not even know what they *really* feel) until some way into the interview when they have reflected on the subject matter and a rapport between interviewer and interviewee has been established. The point is made in a study of health beliefs by Cornwell (1984) who distinguishes between what she terms 'public' and 'private' accounts. A public account is where the interviewee reports what they think will be acceptable to the interviewer – perhaps as a guard against anyone else who may have access to what is said. Public accounts then are framed by the respondent in accordance with what they perceive would be acceptable. Private accounts, by contrast, more closely approximate an authentic record of respondents' subjective beliefs, opinions and attitudes. An example of a public account, derived from interviews conducted with general practitioners and community pharmacists regarding their perceived inter-professional relationships, would be: 'He does his job – I do mine – we get along fine.' This contrasts with a private account: 'I wish he would call me by my first name' (Harding, 1989).

3. *Observational data can supplement transcription data*

Transcripts of recorded interviews in themselves provide information based solely on what was said. When analysing them, researchers therefore attempt to make sense of people's actions, beliefs and behaviour simply on the strength of what they said during the interview. Textual analysis can be reduced to a single dimensional interpretation, whereas it should be used to augment a broader analysis on the basis of the broader physical and social context in which the interview took place. For example, interviews with pharmacists regarding their attitudes to the provision of injecting equipment to drug misusers may usefully be put into the context of the clientele and workload of the pharmacist at the time of the interview. As well as providing a context for the interview transcript, observed information may also supply additional data to be analysed. For example, an interview study of pharmacist –doctor relationships would yield an account of the pharmacist's perception of their relationship. However, if in the course of the interview the researcher witnesses the procedure required of the pharmacist in order to contact the doctor by telephone – for example, initially contacting the receptionist, being put on hold, being told the GP is too busy to speak with him/her and will ring back, or the formality of any exchange – then this observed data, if recorded after the interview in supplementary field notes, may be drawn on to explore how what is verbally reported during interview relates to actual practice.

MAKING SENSE OF RESEARCH EVIDENCE

As highlighted above, the majority of pharmacists, rather than carrying out their own research, will increasingly be required to use research evidence to inform their practice. To do so requires a critical evaluation of published work, whether it is original research or in the form of a systematic review (as produced by the Cochrane Collaboration). Practitioners should be equipped to establish the validity and usefulness of the results. Box 9.3 contains some of the questions which readers of published research might consider in this evaluative process.

Box 9.3 Key questions to ask when evaluating published research

1. Did the study have a clearly focused research question?
2. Were the research methodologies appropriate for the research question?
3. Were the methodologies correctly applied?
4. In review articles, were all the relevant studies included?
5. Are observed differences between groups statistically significant?
6. Were the reported outcomes of the research considered from all relevant perspectives; for instance, if a pharmacy service was evaluated, was the perspective of users, providers and other stakeholders such as general practitioners considered?
7. Are the results generalisable or transferable to the general population?
8. Are the conclusions supported by the results?

Summary

- The research question determines the research methodology
- Social research may be either quantitative or qualitative
- There are dedicated sampling strategies for both qualitative and quantitative methods
- The validity of the results is determined by the robustness of the research instrument
- All research requires consideration of reliability, validity and causality.

Further reading

Review of published social and health services research in pharmacy

Smith, F. (2002) *Research Methods in Pharmacy Practice*, London, Pharmaceutical Press.

Methodological aspects of social surveys

Bowling, A. (2002) *Research Methods in Health* (2nd edn), Buckingham, Open University Press.

Bryman, A. (2001) *Social Research Methods*, Oxford, Oxford University Press.

Gantley, M. (2001) Interviews. In: K.M.G. Taylor and G. Harding (eds) *Pharmacy Practice*, London, Taylor and Francis, pp. 457–472.

Hoinville, G. and Jowell, R. (1983) *Survey Research Practice*, London, Heinemann Educational Books.

Jesson, J. and Pocock, R. (2001) Survey methods. In: K.M.G. Taylor and G. Harding (eds) *Pharmacy Practice*. London, Taylor and Francis, pp. 433–456.

Marsh, C. (1982) *The Survey Method: The Contribution of Surveys to Sociological Explanation*, London, George Allen and Unwin.

Moser, C.A. and Kalton, G. (1983) *Survey Methods in Social Investigation*, Gower, Aldershot.

Silverman, D. (1994) *Interpreting Qualitative Data: Methods for Analysing Talk, Text and Interaction*, London, Sage.

Smith, F. (2001) Focus groups. In: K.M.G. Taylor and G. Harding (eds) *Pharmacy Practice*, London, Taylor and Francis, pp. 473–483.

Tesche, R. (1990) *Qualitative Research: Analysis Types and Software Tools*, London, Falmer Press.

Ethnographic Research

Hammersley, M. and Atkinson, P. (1983) *Ethnography: Principles in Practice*, London, Tavistock Publications.

Research Design

Hakin, C. (1987) *Research Design*, London, Allen and Unwin.

Statistics

Barber, N. (2001) Statistical tests. In: K.M.G. Taylor and G. Harding (eds) *Pharmacy Practice*, London, Taylor and Francis, pp. 493–507.

Jones, D. (2002) *Pharmaceutical Statistics*, London, Pharmaceutical Press.

REFERENCES

Baum, F. (1995) Researching public health: behind the qualitative–quantitative methodological debate. *Social Science and Medicine*, 40, 459–468.

Cook, T.D. and Campbell, D.T. (1979) *Quasi-Experimentation: Design and Analysis Issues for Field Studies*, Chicago, Rand McNally.

Cornwell, J. (1984) *Hard Earned Lives*, London, Tavistock.

Glaser, B.G. and Strauss, A.L. (1967) *The Discovery of Grounded Theory: Strategies for Qualitative Research*, Chicago, Aldine Publishing Company.

Harding, G. (1989) *Pharmaceutical Service Delivery in English Health Centres. Final Report to the Department of Health*, London, University of London.

Jesson, J., Pocock, R., Jepson, M. and Kendall, H. (1994) Consumer readership and views on pharmacy health education literature: a market research survey. *Journal of Social and Administrative Pharmacy*, 11, 29–36.

Krippendorff, K. (1980) *Content Analysis: an Introduction to its Methodology*, London, Sage.

Mills, C.W. (1969) *The Sociological Imagination*, New York, Oxford University Press.

Nichol, M.B., McCombs, J.S., Boghossian, T. and Johnson, K.A. (1992) The impact of patient counselling on over-the-counter drug purchasing behaviour. *Journal of Social and Administrative Pharmacy*, 9, 11–20.

Royal Pharmaceutical Society of Great Britain (1997) *The Report of the Pharmacy Practice Research and Development Task Force: A New Age for Pharmacy Practice Research*, London, Royal Pharmaceutical Society of Great Britain.

Shipman, M. (1988) *The Limitations of Social Research*, London, Longman.

Smith, F. (2002) *Research Methods in Pharmacy Practice*, London, Pharmaceutical Press.

Index

Data Protection Registrar 169
de–skilling 26–7
diagnostic testing 70
disease, definition 38
dispensing 23–5, 70
    robotic 26–7, 123
    supervision of 25, 32
dispensing chemist 119
doctor–patient relationship
    64–8
doctrine of specific aetiology 80
drug abuse, *see* drug misuse
druggist 118
drug misuse 133, 150–1
Durkheim, E. 12–13, 109

efficiency 26
empiricism 159
    abstracted 178
environmental health 136, 141
epidemiology 77, 81–2
ethnicity 96
    health 96–9
ethnography 176
evidence-based medicine 86–7
experimental method 160
expert 16, 116, 122
expert patient 45, 64, 67–8
extemporaneous preparation,
    see compounding
extended role 1, 28–31, 127

first port of call 23
focus group 175
food co-operative 143
Freidson, E. 58–9, 66, 116
French Revolution 12

gender 92, *see* also health
General Household Survey 101
genetically modified food 15,
    44
germ theory 80
Good Pharmacy Practice 132
GP fund holding 84
grounded theory 177

harm minimisation 151

health 37–51, 76–87, 91–110
    commodification 83–5
    definition 81
    ethnicity 96–9
    gender 92–6
    psycho-social circumstances
        108–10
    social class 98–103, 106–8
    social inequalities 91–110
    unemployment 105
Health Action Zones 109
Health Belief Model 50
Health Care in the High Street
    146
Health Development Agency
    135
Health Divide 102, 106, 108
health education 136–40, 144
    approaches 137–9
    definition 136
health and Illness, models
    48–50, 79–81
Health Improvement
    Programme 141
health inequalities 92–110, 134
Health of the Nation 133–4
health policy 110, 133–6, 151
health promotion 70, 131–51
    approaches 142–3
    Beatties' typology 142–3
    definition 139
    drug misuse 139–40, 150–1
    literature 146
    model 139–40
    pharmacy–based 141, 150–1
    self-help group 141
    sociological analyses 143–5
health protection 140
Health and Safety at Work Act
    136
Heart Beat Wales 145
help seeking behaviour 56–72
    triggers 57–8
hospital pharmacy 21–2
Human Genome Project 44
human immunodeficiency
    virus (HIV) 133, 141
hypertension 41, 48–9

hypotension 6
hypothetico-deduction model
172–3

iatrogenesis 83
Illich, I 83
illness 37–51, *see also* health,
symptoms
chronic 45–7, 62
definition 38
prevention 135–6, 140
as a social concept 38–50
illness behaviour 39–44, 149, *see
also* adherence
indeterminate knowledge 117
Industrial Revolution 12
inequalities in health 91–110
informal carers, *see* carers
injecting equipment exchange
151
internal market 83
Internet 122, *see also* World
Wide Web
inter-professional working 124–6
interviews 175–7
depth 177
group 175
non-standardised 177
semi-structured 175
standardised 176
iron cage 14
I/T ratio 117, 127

Johnson, T. 118

lay epidemiology 145
lay health beliefs 47–50, 138
lay health care workers, *see*
carer
lay knowledge 47–50
lay referral system 58–9, 63
lifestyle 132–4, 137–8, 143
limited list 116

Marx, K. 13–14, 100
McDonaldisation 26, 123
McKeown, T. 81–2
measuring health 76–9

Mechanic, D. 40
medical model of health and
disease 79–80
medicalisation 12
medicines
alternative 86
as commodities 84–5
deregulation 85, 123
Pharmacy 120
medicines management 31, 121,
126–7
definition 31
mental illness 133, 141
Methadone 150–1
Migril case 24
Mills, C.W. 8
minor ailment 29–30, 43–4, 56,
69, *see also* illness,
symptoms
modernity 14–15
morbidity rates 78–9
ethnicity 97–9
gender 92–6
shortcomings 79
social class 93–4
mortality rates 77
ethnicity 96–9
gender 92–6, 104
infant 77, 102
neonatal 77
perinatal 77, 102
regional variation 103–4
shortcomings 78
social class 93–4, 102–5
standardised 77
MRSA 83
Mumps, Measles and Rubella
(MMR) vaccine 44
myalgic encephalomyelitis
(ME) 44
myocardial infarction 41
mystification 119

National Health Service (NHS)
83–4, 136, *see also* health
policy
National Pharmaceutical
Association (NPA) 22, 146

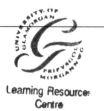